SPECIAL FORCES
FITNESS TRAINING

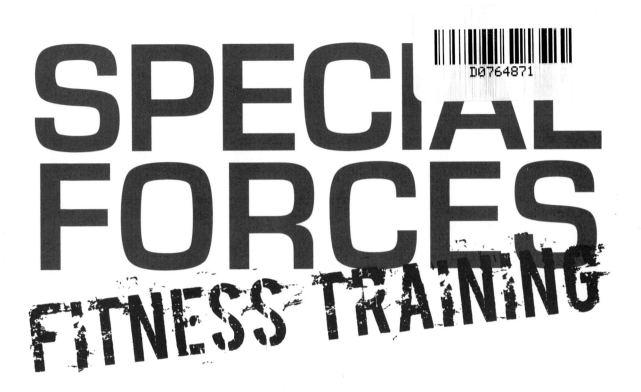

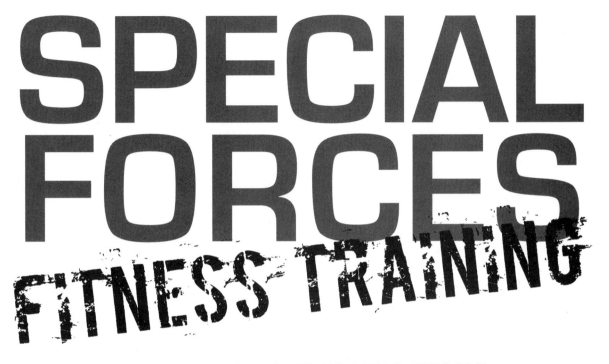

SPECIAL FORCES FITNESS TRAINING

GYM-FREE WORKOUTS TO BUILD MUSCLE AND GET IN ELITE SHAPE

AUGUSTA DEJUAN HATHAWAY

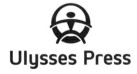

Ulysses Press

Published in the United States by
Ulysses Press
P.O. Box 3440
Berkeley, CA 94703
www.ulyssespress.com

ISBN: 978-1-61243-306-6
Library of Congress Control Number 2013957415

Printed in the United States by Bang Printing

10 9 8 7 6 5 4 3 2 1

Acquisitions: Keith Riegert
Managing editor: Claire Chun
Editor: Lily Chou
Proofreader: Elyce Berrigan-Dunlop
Indexer: Sayre Van Young
Design and layout: what!design @ whatweb.com
Cover photographs: front © NKLRDVC/shutterstock.com; back © Rapt Productions
Interior photographs: © Rapt Productions except on page 17 medicine ball © Sandra Caldwell/shutterstock.com, kettlebell © Stocksnapper/shutterstock.com, weight plate © Kbiros/shutterstock.com, basketball © Aaron Amat/shutterstock.com
Models: Augusta DeJuan Hathaway, Bryan Johnson

Distributed by Publishers Group West

Please Note
This book has been written and published strictly for informational purposes, and in no way should be used as a substitute for actual instruction with qualified professionals. The author and publisher are providing you with information in this work so that you can have the knowledge and can choose, at your own risk, to act on that knowledge. The author and publisher also urge all readers to be aware of their health status and to consult health care professionals before beginning any health program.

I dedicate this book to my mother and sister:
Even though you were with me for a short time, you will forever be in my heart.
Thank you to my father and brother for always encouraging and supporting me.

CONTENTS

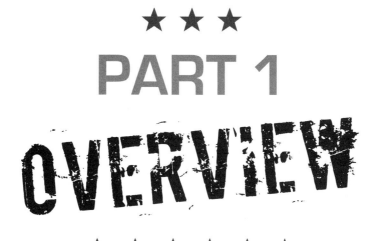

PART 1

OVERVIEW

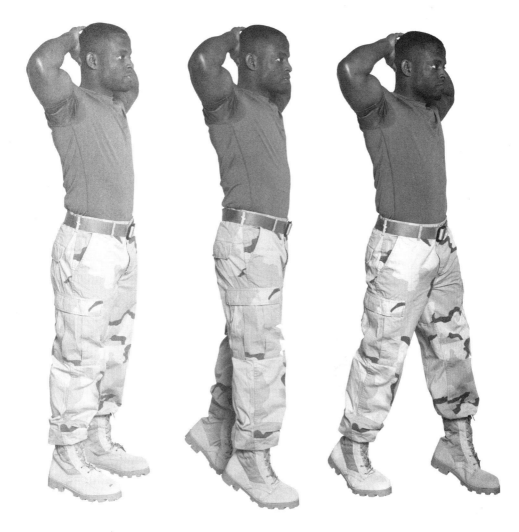

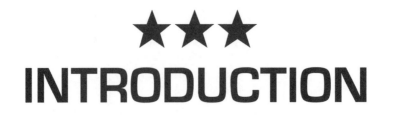

INTRODUCTION

We've all watched action-packed military movies in which an extraordinary soldier carries out a series of heroic acts to successfully complete a mission. Films such as *Rambo*, *Act of Valor*, *Lone Survivor*, *Jarhead* and *The Delta Force* always motivated me to maintain a high level of fitness and also raised my interest in the methods of fitness training special operations groups such as Navy SEALs, Green Berets and Army Rangers partake in. As it turns out, movies only show a portion of the rigorous physical training these soldiers put themselves through daily to become elite soldiers.

Since 2009, I've served as a strength and conditioning specialist for various U.S. military branches. During this time I've been fortunate to have trained some of the most elite soldiers in the world. I created *Special Forces Fitness Training* to offer a different and convenient method for soldiers to perform physical training regardless of their location and deployment status.

Special Forces Fitness Training consists of workouts I created while training personnel of the Army, Air Force, Navy and Marines. Soldiers that utilized this program became stronger, faster and leaner, and also sustained fewer injuries than they did prior to performing this program. How is this possible? Well, just like collegiate or professional athletes, soldiers are required to have speed, agility, strength, balance, endurance, flexibility, quick reflexes and mental toughness. In other words: To be a badass, train like one!

The unique thing about this program is that it not only provides exercise from an athletic spectrum, but also a military spectrum. In this book you'll find 30 different workouts involving the core (abs), upper body, total body, martial arts and much more. No other program offers this combination. Regardless of your gender or fitness level, I can promise that if you push yourself and commit to the program, you'll achieve your desired results.

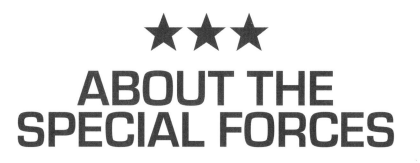

ABOUT THE SPECIAL FORCES

Special operations soldiers are considered the elite representatives of their respective branch of service. The Air Force has the Pararescue, the Navy has its SEAL (Sea, Air, Land) teams, the Marine Corps has Force Reconnaissance (or Force Recon), and the Army has its Green Berets and Ranger units. To be selected for one of these elite teams, one must successfully complete rigorous physical and mental tests under a high level of stress. For example, to become an Air Force Pararescueman, you must be able to swim 50 meters underwater; a Navy SEAL needs to be able to swim 500 meters in 8 to 9 minutes; a Marine Force Recon must be able to tread water for 40 minutes; an Army Ranger needs to run 5 miles in under 40 minutes.

The path to becoming a special ops soldier is not an easy one. Many soldiers train weeks, months and even years to prepare their mind and body for the challenges that they'll encounter during the selection phase. Any special ops solider will tell you that while the physical stress and sacrifice is challenging, successfully completing the selection course makes it all worthwhile.

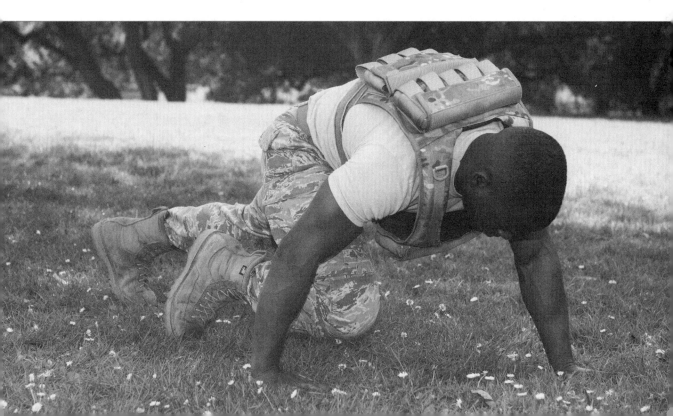

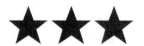

WHY GET SPECIAL FORCES FIT?

Special Forces Fitness Training will forever change how you view military fitness. When many people think of military fitness, push-ups, sit-ups, long runs, weight rooms, and other heavy-duty machinery pop into mind. Yet this program requires only items that can be found in most households and offers a very effective but inexpensive way to achieve a high level of fitness. No gym or cardio equipment is needed to get into tip-top shape.

Over the past ten years I've had the opportunity to train professional and collegiate athletes as well as military personnel. Of those three fields, no training can match the intensity of physical military training. The level of training a soldier has to endure is far more rigorous than any NFL, NBA or combat sport training combined. The prerequisite process to become a part of a special operational forces unit can last for days, weeks and even months, not to mention the daily training events during the selection process that can last anywhere from 1 to 24 hours, and sometimes longer. In order to become a member of the special forces, it takes an internally driven individual who's mentally, physically and emotionally strong.

This is why I've named this program "Special Forces Fitness Training." To endure the challenges of this program, you'll need to be like a special ops soldier: to be driven no matter how challenging the workout may be, to be committed to achieving your fitness goal. This program will not only provide exercises from the athletic realm but also from a military standpoint. There's no other fitness program out there that offers fitness exercises from both a military and athletic approach. So if you're looking for a fitness program that will challenge you, *Special Forces Fitness Training* is the right one for you.

What also makes this program so distinctive is that it's tailored to three levels of fitness: beginner, intermediate and elite. Many fitness programs today only address one group of individuals (the elite level), neglecting everyone else. Many of these programs expect a beginner to initially perform at the elite level. Taking this approach is not only senseless but quickly opens the door to muscular injury due to improper progression. None of us were born with the ability to walk—we first learned to crawl, then walk and then progressed to running. The same concept applies to fitness. No one's born an elite athlete; many elite athletes worked hard daily to reach their peak level of fitness. This program will take you at your initial fitness level and progress you safely to the next level of fitness.

WHAT IF YOU'RE ALREADY IN THE SPECIAL OPERATION FORCES?

If you're already a special forces badass, you may be wondering if *Special Forces Fitness Training* can benefit you. The answer is YES! In fact, I originally created this program as a convenient way for active-duty soldiers to stay in shape while deployed or performing field missions.

The idea came about while preparing a group of soldiers for U.S. Special Forces (Army) and Army Ranger selection. Often we'd begin a strength-and-conditioning cycle but then we'd have to postpone training when the soldiers were deployed or had to focus on field training. More often than not I wouldn't see them for weeks or months at a time.

Upon the continuation of our strength-and-conditioning program, it was as if we were back at square one—all the progress each soldier had gained was lost during that period of not training. In response, I created this program so that soldiers could perform physical training in any location and at any time, utilizing only their issued gear. Immediately the program had a significant impact on soldiers' fitness levels. Their Physical Training (P.T.) test scores dramatically increased, they saw a decrease in body fat percentages and the strength levels they gained did not decrease.

Once I saw the positive effects of this program, I knew it needed to be introduced to any soldier I came across. It has been utilized by special forces personnel of the Air Force, Army, Navy and Marines, active-duty soldiers, reservists and civilians, and the results were all the same. Each individual gained positive fitness results and did so on a daily basis with only military gear. *Special Forces Fitness Training* is probably the most beneficial, productive, inexpensive and effective program any military personnel, or anyone looking to become a part of the military, can partake in. This program will not only change military personnel's perspective about fitness but also the fitness industry.

★★★
FUELING FOR FITNESS

Just as fuel is important for a vehicle, so is food — more importantly, the right foods — for the body. I use this correlation because you have to treat your body as if it's a luxury car. Yes, you can put cheaper-quality gasoline in your car and it will still function, but not at the high level at which your car is capable of performing. The same goes for eating.

Whatever you ingest, good or bad, will have a positive or negative effect on your performance. To get the maximum physical results from this program, it's important to incorporate a nutrition plan consisting of lean meats, fruits, vegetables and water. Limit your intake of fried, processed and other foods that are considered "unhealthy," as well as alcohol, candy and any carbonated drink. If you're not sure which foods you should eat, seek a local nutritionist for assistance. It's true that you are what you eat, so choose wisely!

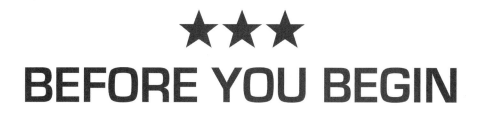

BEFORE YOU BEGIN

Special Forces Fitness Training is for serious people who are serious about being fit. For this reason, you'll have to be mentally driven to push your body beyond its comfort zone. The workouts are very challenging yet doable. Know your level of fitness. If you're at a low level of fitness, remember that the "focus" is on improving your overall fitness. It's not where you start but where you finish! Train hard but safe, follow exercise instructions as described and never sacrifice technique.

Before you jump into the program, however, here are some factors you should consider.

1 If you're unsure about the status of your health, check with your doctor to make sure that you have no physical conditions that may put your health at risk. This applies to anyone planning to undertake this fitness program.

2 To minimize the likelihood of injury, perform each exercise with proper technique as instructed and depicted.

3 For exercises that require equipment you may not have, see the "Equipment" section (page 17).

4 There are going to be days when you experience soreness and your mind is telling you to take a day off. Unless you're injured, push through the soreness. The soreness will decrease as you begin to work out and eventually diminish over the course of a day or two. (Turn to page 16 to learn how to distinguish between good and bad pain.)

5 Do whatever it takes to get that desired level of fitness — work hard, stretch, eat right and get rest!

6 Have fun!

PREVENTING INJURY

To reduce the likelihood of experiencing a muscle injury, it's important to perform a 5- to 10-minute warm-up prior to the workout. This will prepare your muscles by raising your body temperature and allowing adequate blood flow to your muscles. At the completion of any workout, it's important to spend 5 to 10 minutes stretching the muscles you worked. Post-workout is the best time to stretch because your muscles are still warm, which makes muscular flexibility easier to achieve. Stretching after a workout also eliminates lactic acid build-up in the muscles, which causes muscle soreness.

You should also learn the difference between "good pain" and "bad pain." Sometimes after a hard workout, your muscles may be sore the next day and a few days after. This is considered "good pain." The muscle soreness will gradually decrease with rest, recovery and stretching. However, if over the course of a few days your muscle soreness has gone away but you're still experiencing pain or limited range of motion, you may have sustained an injury during your training. This is considered "bad pain." Your injury has damaged a muscle to the point that the muscle cannot properly function as it should. Other common training injuries are joint injuries such as ankle or knee sprains.

Regardless of the degree of your injuries, they should be taken very seriously and you should get treatment immediately. Oftentimes people believe the phrase "no pain no gain" or "work through the pain," but unfortunately this has led many people to believe that unless they're not experiencing some level of physical pain, then the workout SUCKS! In actuality, if you're experiencing pain during your training, there's a possibility that you may have injured yourself. If you're injured, discontinue training, get checked out and take the necessary procedures to heal your injury so you can quickly return to training.

Rest and recovery are highly recommended when participating in this fitness program. Many people hold the misconception that "more is better." This statement is true when proper rest and recovery are included in the training plan. However, neglecting rest and recovery could have a detrimental effect on overall performance. Allow at least 1 to 2 days of complete rest during the week, and allow at least 12 to 24 hours between each workout session. For example, if you perform a workout from 7 to 8 p.m., then your next workout should be performed at 8 a.m. or 8 p.m. the next day. This allows your muscles adequate rest and recovery, which helps maximize muscle growth and strength gains. This also decreases the chances of overtraining.

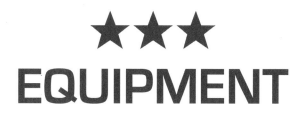

★★★
EQUIPMENT

Although there are plenty of bodyweight movements in this book, some of the exercises require equipment and are demonstrated with military gear. The following is a list of equipment utilized in each section. If you do not have the suggested equipment, simply use one of the recommended substitutions. For example, some of the Core & Stability Exercises require a canteen. If you don't have a canteen, swap in a medicine ball.

WARM-UP EXERCISES: No equipment required for this section.

BALANCE & STABILITY EXERCISES: No equipment required for this section, but the usage of dumbbells is optional.

CORE & STABILITY EXERCISES: Both the military helmet and canteen are utilized in this section.

> **Military Helmet Substitutions:** medicine ball, basketball, 10- to 15-pound dumbbell, 10- to 25-pound weight plate, 10- to 20-pound kettlebell

> **Canteen Substitutions:** medicine ball, 10- to 15-pound dumbbell, 10- to 25-pound weight plate, 10- to 20-pound kettlebell

STRENGTH-TRAINING EXERCISES: This section utilizes the military helmet, body armor vest, combat uniform and sandbag.

> **Military Helmet Substitutions:** medicine ball, basketball, 10- to 15-pound dumbbell, 10- to 25-pound weight plate, 10- to 20-pound kettlebell

> **Body Armor Vest Substitutions:** weight vest, medicine ball, 10- to 15-pound dumbbell, 10- to 25-pound weight plate, 10- to 20-pound kettlebell

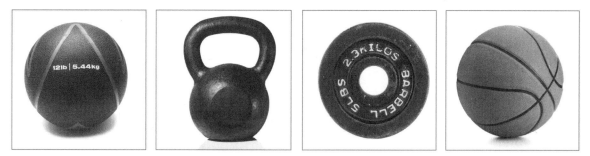

Substitute equipment (left to right): Medicine ball, kettlebell, weight plate, basketball

Combat Uniform Substitutions: towel, rope, bed sheet

Sandbag Substitutions: medicine ball, dumbbells, weight plates, kettlebells

PUSH-UP SERIES: This section utilizes the military helmet.

Military Helmet Substitutions: medicine ball, textbooks, basketball, football

AGILITY, SPEED & PLYOMETRIC EXERCISES: This section utilizes the military helmet and combat uniform.

Combat Uniform Substitutions: towel, rope, bed sheet, cones

Military Helmet Substitutions: medicine ball, textbooks

MARTIAL ARTS CARDIO EXERCISES: No equipment required for this section, but the usage of dumbbells is optional.

FLEXIBILITY EXERCISES: This section utilizes the combat uniform.

Combat Uniform Substitutions: towel, rope, bed sheet

★ ★ ★

PART 2

THE WORKOUTS

★ ★ ★ ★ ★ ★ ★

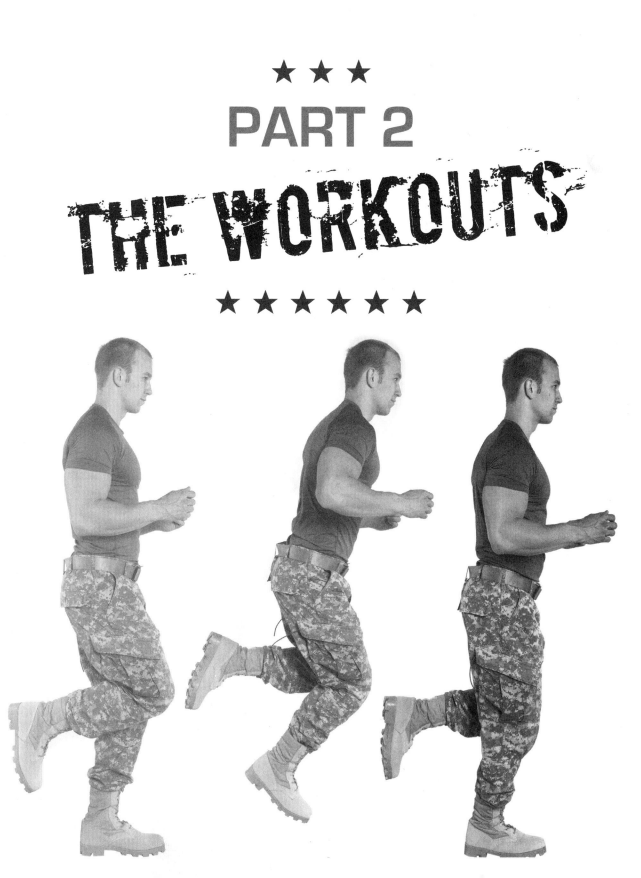

★★★

HOW TO USE THIS BOOK

Regardless of your gender or fitness level, following *Special Forces Fitness Training* is very simple — know your level of fitness and your limits. Whenever I train soldiers, I always tell them to be honest with themselves. Often people have the misconception that if a workout doesn't totally exhaust you, then it must not have been a "good" workout. That belief is not only false but dangerous. Never become so fatigued during a workout that proper exercise technique is no longer utilized. Fatigue and bad exercise form can increase the likelihood of musculoskeletal injury. So keep these in mind when using this or any program: 1) Know your fitness level. 2) *Always* use proper exercise technique. 3) Know your limits.

DETERMINING YOUR WORKOUT PLAN

You'll need to perform the Belasco (page 88) for 5 minutes to determine your initial fitness level. Perform this exercise over a 10-yard distance. Every 10 yards counts as a single repetition (for example, up 10 yards and back 10 yards is the equivalent of two repetitions). Perform as many proper, good-form repetitions as you can in the 5-minute time frame, then consult the chart below to determine your level of fitness. I recommend that you perform this test at least once a month to measure your fitness improvements.

	BEGINNER	INTERMEDIATE	ELITE
FEMALE	6 or less reps	7–9 reps	10 or more reps
MALE	8 or less reps	10–12 reps	15 or more reps

Once you've identified your fitness level, decide how many days a week you prefer to train. Below is a weekly exercise layout chart that presents guidelines for three-, four-, five- and six-day weekly routines. Once you've decided which weekly routine to follow, simply perform the workout for that given day. For example, if you choose to train six days a week, Monday and Friday would consist of total-body workouts; Tuesday and Thursday would be core days;

Wednesday and Sunday would be cardio days, and Saturday would be a recovery day. Activities such as walking, swimming and biking can also be performed on recovery days. I encourage you to create your own personal weekly routine to follow; when doing so, allow at least one day of rest to let your muscles recover.

WEEKLY EXERCISE ROUTINES							
	MONDAY	TUESDAY	WEDNESDAY	THURSDAY	FRIDAY	SATURDAY	SUNDAY
3X A WEEK	Total Body	Rest	Cardio	Rest	Total Body	Rest	Rest
4X A WEEK	Total Body	Core	Rest	Cardio	Rest	Total Body	Rest
5X A WEEK	Total Body	Core	Upper Body	Rest	Upper Body	Cardio	Rest
6X A WEEK	Total Body	Core	Cardio	Core	Total Body	Rest	Cardio

Special Forces Fitness Training provides 30 different workouts so you never have to perform the same workout twice in a month. The workouts are broken down into Total Body, Upper Body, Core (Abs) and Cardio. Throughout the workouts you'll often see different levels ranging from 1 to 3. These levels represent the intensity of the workout (Level 1=low, Level 2=moderate, Level 3=high). Follow the appropriate level based on your 5-minute performance on the Belasco. Remember, it's not where you start but where you finish!

For example:

EXERCISE	LEVEL 1	LEVEL 2	LEVEL 3
Around the Clock	3x3 reps	3x4 reps	3x5 reps
Cross-Body Knee Crunch	3x10 reps	3x12 reps	4x15 reps
Backward Hop	3x10 reps each leg	3x12 reps each leg	4x15 reps each leg
Weaver	3x20 seconds	3x30 seconds	4x40 seconds

BEFORE & AFTER YOUR WORKOUT

Prior to starting any workout routine, perform 3–5 drills from the warm-up section (page 40). It's always important to properly warm up before engaging in high-intensity exercise. A good warm-up raises the body temperature, which allows more flexibility and blood flow to the muscles, reducing the likelihood of encountering an injury during training.

Upon completion of each training session it's also important to perform at least five flexibility exercises (page 147). A lack of flexibility makes muscles short and tight, which ultimately decreases the muscles' range of motion (ROM). Stretching after a workout can drastically increase your ROM since loose and warm muscles make it easier to stretch them. The more range of motion you have, the more mobile you become and the less likely you are to encounter injury.

★ 5 PILLARS

Five Pillars is a total-body workout. To set up the routine, position each station 5 to 20 yards apart from each other. Start at Station 1 and perform the exercise, then sprint to the next station. For example, a man would do 6 sets of 20 Decline Helmet Push-Ups at Station 1, sprint to Station 2 and perform 6 sets of 10 Lunge and Presses per leg before going on to Station 3.

All exercises are performed in body armor.

5 PILLARS		
	EXERCISE	SETS X REPS / DURATION
STATION 1	Decline Helmet Push-Up	*Male:* 6x20 reps	*Female:* 4x10 reps
STATION 2	Static Lunge & Overhead Press	*Male:* 6x10 reps each leg	*Female:* 4x10 reps each leg
STATION 3	Helmet Pull & Tuck	*Male:* 6x30 reps	*Female:* 4x20 reps
STATION 4	Sprint to Back Pedal	*Male:* 6x20 seconds	*Female:* 4x12 seconds
STATION 5	Lateral Crawl	*Male:* 6x20 reps	*Female:* 4x10 reps

★ 4 CORNERS

Four Corners is a total-body workout. Set up each corner a minimum of 5 yards apart from each other. Start at Corner 1 and perform the exercise, then sprint to the next corner. For example, a man would perform 20 sandbag squat and presses at Corner 1 before sprinting to Corner 2 to do 40 jumping jacks. Once he finishes all four corners, he repeats the series 3 more times for a total of 4.

For rounds 1 and 2, male duration is 6 minutes, rest 4 minutes; female duration is 4 minutes, rest 3 minutes. For round 3, male duration is 8 minutes, rest 5 minutes; female duration is 6 minutes, rest 5 minutes. For round 4, male duration is 10 minutes, rest 6 minutes; female duration is 6 minutes, rest 6 minutes.

4 CORNERS		
	EXERCISE	SETS X REPS / DURATION
CORNER 1	Sandbag Squat & Press	*Male:* 4x20 reps	*Female:* 3x10 reps
CORNER 2	Jumping Jacks	*Male:* 4x40 reps	*Female:* 4x20 reps
CORNER 3	Cross-Body Crunch	*Male:* 4x30 reps	*Female:* 4x20 reps
CORNER 4	Helmet Plyo Push-Up	*Male:* 4x10 reps each arm	*Female:* 4x6 reps each arm

★ KING OF THE JUNGLE

King of the Jungle is a total-body workout. Choose a level that will push you! Perform the exercises in the order in which they're listed, and perform all sets and repetitions before moving on to the next exercise. When performing the shadow boxing and shadow kickboxing exercises, you may choose any boxing and kickboxing combination from the Martial Arts Cardio section (page 135). This workout is dedicated to the men and women of the U.S. Navy, and especially to Kaneohe Marine Naval Base, Hawaii: "Honor, Courage, Commitment."

KING OF THE JUNGLE			
EXERCISE	SETS X REPS / DURATION		
	LEVEL 1	LEVEL 2	LEVEL 3
3 Hops & Reach	3x3 reps each leg	3x4 reps each leg	3x5 reps each leg
Alternating V	3x10 reps	3x10 reps	3x10 reps
Statue of Liberty	3x10 reps each leg	3x12 reps each leg	4x15 reps each leg
Crunch Extension	3x10 reps	3x12 reps	4x15 reps
Body Armor Squat to Press	3x20 seconds	3x30 seconds	3x40 seconds
Push-Up with Knee Tuck	3x20 seconds	3x30 seconds	3x40 seconds
Single-Arm Sandbag Swing	3x10 reps each arm	3x12 reps each arm	4x15 reps each arm
Overhead Sandbag Press	3x10 reps	3x12 reps	4x15 reps
Sandbag Walk	1x2 minutes	1x3 minutes	1x5 minutes
Push-Up to Shuffle	3x20 seconds	3x30 seconds	4x1 minute
Mountain Climber	3x20 seconds	3x30 seconds	4x1 minute
Sandbag Upright Row	3x10 reps	3x12 reps	4x15 reps
Shuffle & Touch	3x20 seconds	3x30 seconds	4x1 minute
Shadow Kickboxing	1x2 minutes	1x5 minutes	1x8 minutes
The Belasco	1x2 minutes	1x3 minutes	1x4 minutes

★ THE CROC

The Croc is a total-body workout. Choose a level that will push you! Perform the exercises in the order in which they're listed, and perform all sets and repetitions before moving on to the next exercise. This workout is dedicated to the men and women of the U.S. Air Force: *"Aim High…Fly-Fight-Win."*

THE CROC			
EXERCISE	LEVEL 1	LEVEL 2	LEVEL 3
Around the Clock	3x3 reps	3x4 reps	3x5 reps
Cross-Body Knee Crunch	3x10 reps	3x12 reps	4x15 reps
Backward Hop	3x10 reps each leg	3x12 reps each leg	4x15 reps each leg
Weaver	3x20 seconds	3x30 seconds	4x40 seconds
Sandbag Swing	3x20 seconds	3x30 seconds	4x40 seconds
360° Bear Crawl	3x20 seconds	3x30 seconds	4x40 seconds
Sandbag Squat & Press	3x10 reps	3x12 reps	4x15 reps
Quick Shuffle & Jump	3x35 seconds	3x45 seconds	4x1 minute
Push-Up with Shoulder Tap	3x20 seconds	3x30 seconds	4x40 seconds
Pull-Apart	3x10 reps	3x12 reps	4x15 reps
Bent-Over Row	3x20 seconds	3x30 seconds	4x1 minute
Sandbag Biceps Curl	3x20 seconds	3x30 seconds	4x1 minute

★ WAR BUDDY

War Buddy is a total-body workout performed with a partner. Choose a level that will push you! Perform the exercises in the order in which they're listed, and perform all sets and repetitions before moving on to the next exercise. For the shadow kickboxing exercise, you may choose any punching and kicking combination from the Martial Arts Cardio section (page 135).

WAR BUDDY			
EXERCISE	LEVEL 1	LEVEL 2	LEVEL3
Wheel Barrow Push-Up	3x10 yards	4x20 yards	5x30 yards
Partner Pull-Up	3x10 reps	3x12 reps	4x15 reps
Around the World	3x30 seconds	3x45 seconds	3x1 minute
Helmet Press	3x10 reps	3x12 reps	4x15 reps
Combat Uniform Partner Sprints	3x20 seconds	3x30 seconds	4x30 seconds
Double-Leg Curl	3x10 reps	3x12 reps	4x15 reps
Combat Uniform Backpedal	3x10 yards	4x20 yards	5x30 yards
Overhead Knee Tuck	3x30 seconds	3x45 seconds	3x1 minute
Neck Strengthening 1	1x20 seconds each direction	2x20 seconds each direction	2x25 seconds each direction
Neck Strengthening 2	1x20 seconds each direction	2x20 seconds each direction	2x25 seconds each direction
Shadow Kickboxing	1x6 minutes	1x12 minutes	1x15 minutes

★ GREAT WHITE

The Great White is a total-body workout. Choose a level that will push you! Perform the exercises in the order in which they're listed, completing all sets and repetitions before moving on to the next exercise.

EXERCISE	SETS X REPS		
	Level 1	Level 2	Level 3
Statue of Liberty	3x8 reps	3x10 reps	3x12 reps
Incline Plank Hold	3x30 seconds	3x35 seconds	3x1 minute
Reach & Hold	3x30 seconds	3x35 seconds	3x1 minute
Twist & Reach	3x12 reps	3x15 reps	3x20 reps
Single-Arm Sandbag Swing	3x8 reps	3x12 reps	4x12 reps
Body Armor Bear Crawl	3x15 yards	3x20 yards	4x35 yards
Mountain Topper	3x30 seconds	3x35 seconds	4x1 minute
10-yard Sprint to 360° Shuffle	3x35 seconds	3x45 seconds	4x1 minute
Body Armor Static Lunge & Overhead Press	3x10 yards	3x15 yards	4x20 yards
Stationary Switch Feet	3x30 seconds	3x35 seconds	4x1 minute
Sandbag Push Toss	3x8 reps	3x12 reps	4x12 reps
Quick Sprint	3x20 seconds	3x25 seconds	4x30 seconds
The Belasco	3x35 seconds	3x45 seconds	4x1 minute
10-yard Sprint to Toe Tap	3x45 seconds	4x1 minute	4x1 minute

Table heading: GREAT WHITE

★ THE HITMAN

The Hitman is a very intense total-body workout that consists of 3 rounds. Choose a level that will push you! Each round is performed for a time limit before moving on to the next round. For example, in Round 1 at Level 3, perform 10 repetitions of Sandbag Push-Up to Squat Toss, 10 repetitions of Twist & Reach, and 10 repetitions of Crossover Push-Up. Repeat each exercise for the duration of the round. At the end of 10 minutes, you receive a 5-minute rest.

THE HITMAN	
EXERCISE	REPS
ROUND 1	
Sandbag Push-Up to Squat Toss	10 reps
Twist & Reach	10 reps
Crossover Push-Up	10 reps
Duration — *Level 1:* 3 minute | *Level 2:* 5 minutes | *Level 3:* 10 minutes	
Rest — *Level 1:* 1 minute | *Level 2:* 2 minutes | *Level 3:* 5 minutes	

ROUND 2	
Alternating Upright Row	10 reps
Quick Shuffle	10 reps
Combat Uniform Row	10 reps
Duration — *Level 1:* 3 minute | *Level 2:* 5 minutes | *Level 3:* 10 minutes Rest — *Level 1:* 1 minute | *Level 2:* 2 minutes | *Level 3:* 5 minutes	
ROUND 3	
10-yard Body Armor Bear Crawl	2 trips
10-yard Body Armor Crab Walk & Kick	2 trips
Duration — *Level 1:* 3 minute | *Level 2:* 5 minutes | *Level 3:* 10 minutes Rest — *Level 1:* 1 minute | *Level 2:* 2 minutes | *Level 3:* 5 minutes	

★ THE GRIZZLY

The Grizzly is a total-body workout. Choose a level that will push you! Perform the exercises in the order in which they're listed, completing all sets and repetitions before moving on to the next exercise. For the shadow boxing exercise, you may choose any punching combination from the Martial Arts Cardio section (page 135). This workout is dedicated to the men and women of Ft. Bragg, North Carolina.

THE GRIZZLY			
EXERCISES	SETS X REPS / DURATION		
	Level 1	Level 2	Level 3
3 Hops & Reach	3x8 reps	3x10 reps	3x12 reps
Helmet Toss & Catch	3x15 reps	3x20 reps	3x30
Single-Leg 180 Turn	3x8 reps	3x10 reps	3x12 reps
Decline Plank Hold	3x30 seconds	3x35 seconds	3x1 minute
Single-Arm Sandbag Swing	3x8 reps	3x12 reps	4x12 reps
Body Armor Bear Crawl	3x15 yards	3x20 yards	4x35 yards
Inchworm to Push-Up	3x8 reps	3x10 reps	4x12 reps
Squat Jump	3x8 reps	3x10 reps	4x15 reps
Combat Uniform Row	3x8 reps	3x10 reps	4x15 reps
Shuffle Touch	3x30 seconds	3x35 seconds	3x1 minute
Crossover Push-Up	3x20 seconds	3x25 seconds	4x30 seconds
Stationary Sprint	3x20 seconds	3x25 seconds	4x30 seconds
Double Trouble	3x35 seconds	3x45 seconds	4x1 minute
Shadow Box	1x10 minutes	1x15 minutes	1x20 minutes

★ BUILDING THE FOUNDATION

Building the Foundation is a total-body workout. Perform the exercises in the order in which they're listed, completing all sets and repetitions before moving on to the next exercise.

BUILDING THE FOUNDATION	
EXERCISE	SETS X REPS / DURATION
Combat Uniform Single-Leg Squat	*Male:* 3x15 reps	*Female:* 2x6 reps
Helmet Jumpover	*Male:* 3x15 reps	*Female:* 2x10 reps
Sandbag Squat	*Male:* 3x15 reps	*Female:* 2x6 reps
Reach & Pull	*Male:* 3x15 reps	*Female:* 2x8 reps
Quick Shuffle & Jump	*Male:* 3x15 reps	*Female:* 2x6 reps
Push Kick	*Male:* 3x12 reps	*Female:* 2x8 reps
Around the Clock	*Male:* 3x15 reps	*Female:* 2x6 reps
Seated Punch	*Male:* 3x40 seconds	*Female:* 2x30 seconds
Sprint to 360° Shuffle	*Male:* 3x35 seconds	*Female:* 3x20 seconds

★ STICKING WITH THE BASICS

Sticking with the Basics is an upper-body workout. Perform the exercises in the order in which they're listed, completing all sets and repetitions before moving on to the next exercise.

STICKING WITH THE BASICS	
EXERCISE	SETS X REPS / DURATION
Close-Grip Canteen Push-Up	*Male:* 3x15 reps	*Female:* 2x6 reps
Shin Grab	*Male:* 3x15 reps	*Female:* 2x10 reps
Decline Helmet Push-Up	*Male:* 3x15 reps	*Female:* 2x6 reps
Alternating Vs	*Male:* 3x15 reps	*Female:* 2x8 reps
Push-Up with Knee Tuck	*Male:* 3x15 reps	*Female:* 2x6 reps
Decline Pull & Tuck	*Male:* 3x12 reps	*Female:* 2x8 reps
Helmet Plyo Push-Up	*Male:* 3x15 reps	*Female:* 2x6 reps
Seated Punch	*Male:* 3x40 seconds	*Female:* 2x30 seconds
Explosive Plyo Push-Up	*Male:* 3x15 reps	*Female:* 2x6 reps

★ UPPER BODY I

Upper Body I and Upper Body II are two options for a challenging upper-body workout. For both programs, perform the exercises in the order in which they're listed, completing all sets and repetitions before moving on to the next exercise.

UPPER BODY I	
EXERCISE	SETS X REPS / DURATION
Sandbag Overhead Press	*Male:* 5x20 reps	*Female:* 3x10 reps
Combat Uniform Single Row	*Male:* 5x15 reps	*Female:* 3x10 reps
Offset Hand Push-Up	*Male:* 5x10 reps each side	*Female:* 3x6 reps each side
Punch Combination #5	*Male:* 5x5 minutes	*Female:* 3x3 minutes
Incline Plank Hold	*Male:* 5x1 minute	*Female:* 3x45 seconds
Sandbag Row	*Male:* 5x20 reps	*Female:* 3x12 reps

★ UPPER BODY II

UPPER BODY II	
EXERCISE	SETS X REPS / DURATION
Sandbag Chest Press	*Male:* 5x15 reps	*Female:* 3x10 reps
Overhead Knee Tuck	*Male:* 5x15 reps	*Female:* 3x10 reps
Combat Uniform T-Row	*Male:* 5x10 reps each side	*Female:* 3x6 reps each side
Decline Plank Hold	*Male:* 5x1 minute	*Female:* 3x45 seconds
Half Push-Up	*Male:* 5x20 reps	*Female:* 3x12 reps
Mountain Toppers	*Male:* 5x1 minute	*Female:* 3x45 seconds
Punch Combination #1	*Male:* 5x3 minutes	*Female:* 3x2 minutes
Crossover Push-Up	*Male:* 5x30 seconds	*Female:* 3x20 seconds
Sandbag Curl	*Male:* 5x15 reps	*Female:* 3x10 reps

★ GET A GRIP

Get a Grip is an intense upper-body workout that consists of 3 rounds. Perform the exercises in the order in which they're listed, completing all sets and repetitions before moving on to the next exercise. Take the prescribed rest before starting the next round.

GET A GRIP	
EXERCISE	**SETS X REPS / DURATION**
ROUND 1	
Sandbag Walk	*Male:* 3 minutes | *Female:* 2 minutes
Sandbag Isolation Hold	*Male:* 1 minute | *Female:* 25 seconds
Sandbag Biceps Curl	*Male:* 10 reps | *Female:* 6 reps
Alternating Lunge or Air Squat	*Male:* 30 reps | *Female:* 20 reps
Recovery — *Male:* 3 minutes | *Female:* 2 minutes	
ROUND 2	
Sandbag Walk	*Male:* 5 minutes | *Female:* 3 minutes
Sandbag Isolation Hold	*Male:* 2 minutes | *Female:* 30 seconds
Sandbag Biceps Curl	*Male:* 15 reps | *Female:* 10 reps
Alternating Lunge or Air Squat	*Male:* 60 reps | *Female:* 40 reps
Recovery — *Male:* 3 minutes | *Female:* 1:30 minutes	
ROUND 3	
Sandbag Walk	*Male:* 7 minutes | *Female:* 5 minutes
Sandbag Isolation Hold	*Male:* 2 minutes | *Female:* 50 seconds
Sandbag Biceps Curl	*Male:* 20 reps | *Female:* 12 reps
Alternating Lunge or Air Squat	*Male:* 100 reps | *Female:* 60 reps
Workout Completed	

★ THE FEW

The Few is a very intense total-body workout that consists of 3 rounds. Each round is performed within a given time limit. For example, Round 1 is performed for 6 continuous minutes. At the completion of each round, take a prescribed rest before starting the next round (for Round 1, you'd recover for 4 minutes before starting Round 2). This workout is dedicated to the men and women of the U.S. Marine Corps: HOORAH!

THE FEW	
EXERCISE	**REPS IN A SET**
Body Armor Air Squat	*Male:* 30 reps | *Female:* 20 reps
Lateral Crawl	*Male:* 20 yards | *Female:* 10 yards
Plank with Knee Tuck	*Male:* 1 minute | *Female:* 45 seconds
Push Kick	*Male:* 20 reps each leg | *Female:* 15 reps each leg

	DURATION	**RECOVERY TIME**
ROUND 1	as many sets as possible in 6 minutes	4 minutes
ROUND 2	as many sets as possible in 8 minutes	5 minutes
ROUND 3	as many sets as possible in 10 minutes	Workout Completed

★ THE SILVERBACK

Choose a level that will push you in this total-body workout! Perform the exercises in the order in which they're listed, completing all sets and repetitions before moving on to the next exercise. This workout is dedicated to the U.S. Army, especially the men and women of the 150th and 119th Infantry Battalions at Ft. Benning, Georgia: "This We'll Defend."

THE SILVERBACK			
EXERCISE	**SETS X REPS / DURATION**		
	Level 1	**Level 2**	**Level 3**
Lateral Hop	3x8 reps	3x10 reps	3x12 reps
Overhead Knee Tuck	3x30 seconds	3x35 seconds	3x1 minute
Single-Leg Backward Hop	3x30 seconds	3x35 seconds	3x1 minute
Crunch Extension	3x12 reps	3x15 reps	3x20 reps
Backward Sandbag Toss	3x8 reps	3x12 reps	4x12 reps
Body Armor Alternating Lunge	3x15 yards	3x20 yards	4x35 yards
Helmet 6-Count Push-Up	3x30 seconds	3x35 seconds	4x1 minute
4 Toe Taps to 360° Shuffle	3x35 seconds	3x45 seconds	4x1 minute
Double Trouble	3x10 yards	3x15 yards	4x20 yards
Helmet Jumpover	3x30 seconds	3x35 seconds	4x1 minute
Sandbag Push Toss	3x8 reps	3x12 reps	4x12 reps
Sprint & Touch	3x20 seconds	3x30 seconds	4x1 minute

★ WARRIORS

Warriors is a total-body workout performed with a partner. Perform the exercises in the order in which they're listed, completing all sets and repetitions before moving on to the next exercise.

WARRIORS	
EXERCISE	**SETS X REPS / DURATION**
Buddy Carry	*Male:* 4x40 yards | *Female:* 3x20 yards
Partner Pull-Up	*Male:* 4x10 yards | *Female:* 3x8 yards
Sandbag Twist & Toss	*Male:* 4x10 reps | *Female:* 3x8 reps
Push-Up to Shuffle	*Male:* 4x20 seconds | *Female:* 3x10 seconds
Wheel Barrow Push-Up	*Male:* 4x20 yards | *Female:* 3x10 yards
Sprint & Touch	*Male:* 4x20 seconds | *Female:* 3x10 seconds
Helmet Press	*Male:* 4x30 reps | *Female:* 3x20 reps

★ THE D-TRAIN CHALLENGE

The D-Train Challenge is an intense total-body workout that consists of 4 rounds. Perform the exercises in the order in which they're listed, completing all sets and repetitions before moving on to the next exercise. At the completion of each round, take a prescribed break before starting the next round. This workout is dedicated to every solider that I've had the opportunity to train. Always know that no one knows how to kick your butt like the D-Train!

THE D-TRAIN CHALLENGE	
EXERCISE	**REPS/DURATION**
Sandbag Push Toss	*Male:* 6 reps | *Female:* 3 reps
Crab Walk & Kick	*Male:* 15 yards | *Female:* 10 yards
10-yard Sprint & Touch	*Male:* x2 trips | *Female:* x1 trip
Backward Toss	*Male:* 6 reps | *Female:* 3 reps
Cross-Body Crunch	*Male:* 20 reps | *Female:* 12 reps
Body Armor Bear Crawl	*Male:* 20 yards | *Female:* 10 yards

	DURATION	RECOVERY TIME
ROUND 1	*Male:* 8 minutes | *Female:* 5 minutes	3–5 minutes
ROUND 2	*Male:* 10 minutes | *Female:* 6 minutes	4–6 minutes
ROUND 3	*Male:* 8 minutes | *Female:* 5 minutes	3–5 minutes
ROUND 4	*Male:* 10 minutes | *Female:* 6 minutes	10 minutes

★ CORE WORKOUT I

Core Workouts I, II, III and IV are designed to improve the muscles of the abdominal region. For all four core workout programs, perform the exercises in the order in which they're listed, completing all sets and repetitions before moving on to the next exercise.

CORE WORKOUT I	
EXERCISE	SETS X REPS / DURATION
Shin Grab	*Male:* 5x1 minute | *Female:* 5x30 seconds
Decline Plank Hold	*Male:* 5x1 minute | *Female:* 6x30 seconds
Seated Punch	*Male:* 5x1 minute | *Female:* 6x30 seconds
Helmet Oblique Twist	*Male:* 5x1 minute | *Female:* 6x30 seconds
Crunch Extension	*Male:* 5x1 minute | *Female:* 6x30 seconds

★ CORE WORKOUT II

CORE WORKOUT II	
EXERCISE	SETS X REPS / DURATION
Alternating V	*Male:* 5x1 minute | *Female:* 5x30 seconds
Elevated Plank	*Male:* 5x1 minute | *Female:* 6x30 seconds
Weaver	*Male:* 5x1 minute | *Female:* 6x30 seconds
Around the World	*Male:* 5x1 minute | *Female:* 6x35 seconds
Twist & Reach	*Male:* 5x1 minute | *Female:* 6x30 seconds

★ CORE WORKOUT III

CORE WORKOUT III	
EXERCISE	SETS X REPS / DURATION
Cross-Body Crunch	*Male:* 5x1 minute | *Female:* 5x30 seconds
Overhead Knee Tuck	*Male:* 5x1 minute | *Female:* 6x30 seconds
Alternating Leg Extension	*Male:* 5x1 minute | *Female:* 6x30 seconds
Shin Grab	*Male:* 5x1 minute | *Female:* 6x35 seconds
Twist & Reach	*Male:* 5x1 minute | *Female:* 6x30 seconds

★ CORE WORKOUT IV

CORE WORKOUT IV	
EXERCISE	SETS X REPS / DURATION
Crunch Extension	*Male:* 5x1 minute | *Female:* 5x30 seconds
Decline Plank Hold	*Male:* 5x1 minute | *Female:* 6x30 seconds
Helmet Toss & Catch	*Male:* 5x1 minute | *Female:* 6x30 seconds
Helmet Oblique Twist	*Male:* 5x1 minute | *Female:* 6x30 seconds
Seated Punch	*Male:* 5x1 minute | *Female:* 6x30 seconds

★ SPEED WORKOUT I

Speed Workouts I, II, III, IV, V and VI are intense cardio programs that provide a great way to improve running speed, change of direction, cardiovascular and muscle endurance. For all six programs, perform the exercises in the order in which they're listed, completing all sets and repetitions before moving on to the next exercise. Since the main objective of this workout is speed improvement, perform each drill with maximum effort.

SPEED WORKOUT I	
EXERCISE	SETS X REPS / DURATION
Arm Swing	*Male:* 5x40 seconds | *Female:* 5x30 seconds
Shuffle & Touch	*Male:* 6x20 seconds | *Female:* 6x15 seconds
Stationary Top to Bottom	*Male:* 6x20 seconds | *Female:* 6x15 seconds
Lateral Hop	*Male:* 6x20 seconds | *Female:* 6x15 seconds
Sprint to 360° Shuffle	*Male:* 6x20 seconds | *Female:* 6x15 seconds

★ SPEED WORKOUT II

SPEED WORKOUT II	
EXERCISE	SETS X REPS / DURATION
Arm Swing	*Male:* 5x40 seconds | *Female:* 5x30 seconds
Over the Hill	*Male:* 6x20 seconds | *Female:* 6x15 seconds
Quick Shuffle & Jump	*Male:* 6x20 seconds | *Female:* 6x15 seconds
Sprint to Toe Taps	*Male:* 6x20 seconds | *Female:* 6x15 seconds
4 Toe Taps to 360° Shuffle	*Male:* 6x20 seconds | *Female:* 6x15 seconds

★ SPEED WORKOUT III

SPEED WORKOUT III	
EXERCISE	SETS X REPS / DURATION
Arm Swing	*Male:* 5x40 seconds | *Female:* 5x30 seconds
Helmet Toe Tap	*Male:* 6x20 seconds | *Female:* 6x15 seconds
Push-Up & Shuffle	*Male:* 6x20 seconds | *Female:* 6x15 seconds
Quick Shuffle & Jump	*Male:* 6x20 seconds | *Female:* 6x15 seconds
Sprint to Backpedal	*Male:* 6x20 seconds | *Female:* 6x15 seconds
Helmet Jumpover	*Male:* 6x20 seconds | *Female:* 6x15 seconds

★ SPEED WORKOUT IV

SPEED WORKOUT IV	
EXERCISE	SETS X REPS / DURATION
Arm Swing	*Male:* 5x40 seconds | *Female:* 5x30 seconds
360° Shuffle	*Male:* 6x20 seconds | *Female:* 6x15 seconds
Quick Shuffle	*Male:* 6x20 seconds | *Female:* 6x15 seconds
Sprint & Touch	*Male:* 6x20 seconds | *Female:* 6x15 seconds
Helmet Jumpover	*Male:* 6x20 seconds | *Female:* 6x15 seconds
360° Bear Crawl	*Male:* 6x20 seconds | *Female:* 6x15 seconds

★ SPEED WORKOUT V

SPEED WORKOUT V	
EXERCISE	SETS X REPS / DURATION
Arm Swing	*Male:* 5x40 seconds | *Female:* 5x30 seconds
High Knees Forward & Backward	*Male:* 6x40 seconds | *Female:* 6x20 seconds
Partner Combat Uniform Sprint	*Male:* 6x20 seconds | *Female:* 6x15 seconds
Stepover Forward & Backward	*Male:* 6x40 seconds | *Female:* 6x20 seconds
Stationary Sprint	*Male:* 6x20 seconds | *Female:* 6x15 seconds
Alternating Lunge	*Male:* 6x40 seconds | *Female:* 6x30 seconds

★ SPEED WORKOUT VI

SPEED WORKOUT VI	
EXERCISE	**SETS X REPS / DURATION**
Arm Swing	*Male:* 5x40 seconds	*Female:* 5x30 seconds
Skip & Clap	*Male:* 6x40 seconds	*Female:* 6x20 seconds
Sprint to Backpedal	*Male:* 6x40 seconds	*Female:* 6x20 seconds
Crunch Extension	*Male:* 6x20 seconds	*Female:* 6x15 seconds
Ankle Tap	*Male:* 6x40 seconds	*Female:* 6x20 seconds
Body Armor Air Squat	*Male:* 6x20 seconds	*Female:* 6x15 seconds
Jump Squat	*Male:* 6x40 seconds	*Female:* 6x30 seconds

★ GASSER I

Gasser I and II are intense cardio workouts that provide a great way to improve change of direction and cardiovascular and muscle endurance. For both programs, perform the exercises in the order in which they're listed, completing all sets and repetitions before moving on to the next exercise. In addition, perform drills with maximum effort.

GASSER I	
EXERCISE	**SETS X REPS / DURATION**
Sprint & Touch	*Male:* 4x25 seconds	*Female:* 3x15 seconds
Helmet Toe Tap	*Male:* 4x25 seconds	*Female:* 3x15 seconds
Shuffle & Touch	*Male:* 4x25 seconds	*Female:* 3x15 seconds
Arm Swing	*Male:* 4x25 seconds	*Female:* 3x15 seconds
Jump Squat	*Male:* 4x25 seconds	*Female:* 3x15 seconds
Punch & Kick Combo #1	*Male:* 4x2 minutes	*Female:* 3x1 minute

★ GASSER II

GASSER II	
EXERCISE	**SETS X REPS / DURATION**
Sprint to Backpedal	*Male:* 5x25 seconds	*Female:* 5x15 seconds
Helmet Toe Tap	*Male:* 5x25 seconds	*Female:* 5x15 seconds
Stationary Sprint	*Male:* 5x25 seconds	*Female:* 5x15 seconds
Punch & Kick Combo #2	*Male:* 4x25 seconds	*Female:* 3x15 seconds
Jumping Jacks	*Male:* 4x25 seconds	*Female:* 3x15 seconds
Punch & Kick Combo #2	*Male:* 4x2 minutes	*Female:* 3x1 minute

★ HEART OF A CHAMPION

Heart of a Champion is an intense total-body cardio workout that consists of 6 rounds. For each round, the time duration and the number of push-up/sit-ups decreases. For example, Round 1 consists of 6 minutes of shadow kickboxing versus 3 minutes in Round 3. The recovery time also changes after Round 3. For Rounds 1-3, you receive a 2 to 3-minute recovery; in Rounds 4–6, you get a 1-minute recovery. This workout is dedicated to the men and women serving in the U.S. Armed Forces, for you truly have a Heart of a Champion.

HEART OF A CHAMPION	
EXERCISE	SETS X REPS / DURATION
ROUND 1	
Shadow Kickbox	6 minutes
Alternating V	*Male:* 1x60 reps	*Female:* 1x40 reps
Recovery: 2 minutes	
ROUND 2	
Shadow Kickbox	5 minutes
Knee-Tuck Push-Up	*Male:* 1x50 reps	*Female:* 1x30 reps
Recovery: 2 minutes	
ROUND 3	
Shadow Kickbox	4 minutes
Alternating V	*Male:* 1x40 reps	*Female:* 1x20 reps
Recovery: 2 minutes	
ROUND 4	
Shadow Kickbox	3 minutes
Knee-Tuck Push-Up	*Male:* 1x30 reps	*Female:* 1x20 reps
Recovery: 1 minute	
ROUND 5	
Shadow Kickbox	2 minutes
Push & Sit-Up	*Male:* 1x20 reps	*Female:* 1x10 reps
Recovery: 1 minute	
ROUND 6	
Shadow Kickbox	1 minute
Push & Sit-Up	*Male:* 1x10 reps	*Female:* 1x10 reps
Workout Completed	

★ ★ ★

PART 3

EXERCISES

★ ★ ★ ★ ★ ★ ★

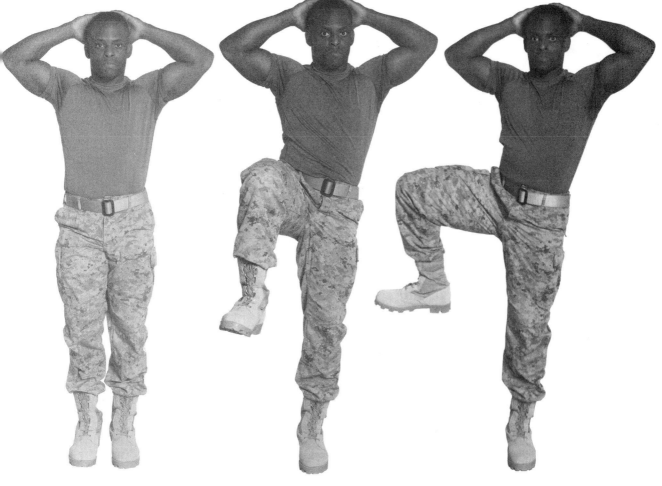

★ WARM-UP SERIES ★

This section is designed to increase blood flow to the muscles of the upper and lower extremities prior to engaging in high-intensity training. Perform 3–5 drills until your muscles become loose and warm.

★ BALLERINA WALK

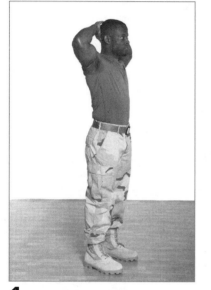 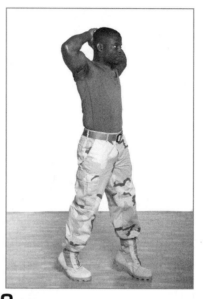

1 Stand upright with your hands placed on top of your head.

2 Lift your heels off the ground and walk on the balls of your feet to the set destination. Don't allow your heels to contact the ground at any point during this drill.

★ SHIN HUG

This drill can be done in place or while moving forward.

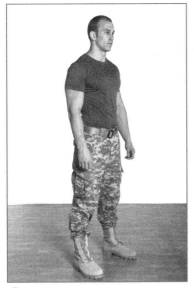

1 Stand upright.

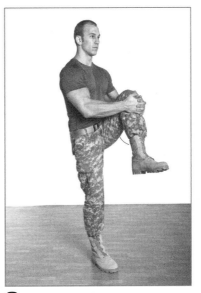

2 Bend one knee, grab your shin with both hands and pull your knee in an upward motion toward your chest.

Alternate legs.

★ QUAD PULL & REACH

This drill can be done in place or while moving forward.

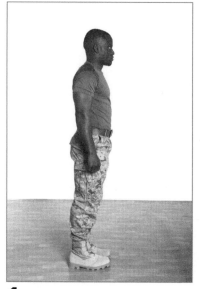

1 Stand upright.

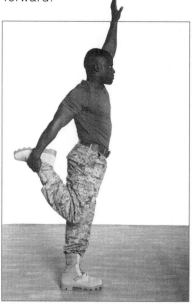

2 Bend your right leg and bring your right heel to your butt. With your right hand, reach behind to grab your right foot. Take your left hand up to the ceiling.

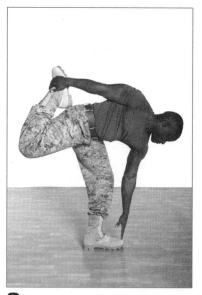

3 Bend at the waist, reach forward with your left hand and touch your left toe.

Alternate legs.

★ WALKING STRAIGHT-LEG KICK

This drill can be done in place or while moving forward.

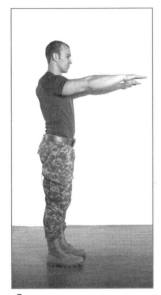

1 Stand upright with your feet together and arms extended forward.

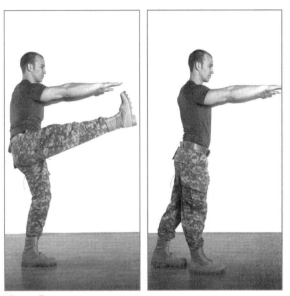

2-3 With your right leg, kick upward until your right toes reach your hands and then step forward.

Alternate legs.

★ STEPOVER

This drill can be done in place or while moving forward and backward.

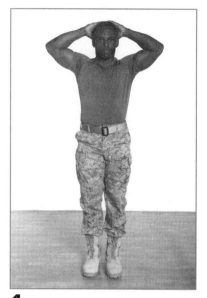

1 Stand upright with your hands placed on top of your head.

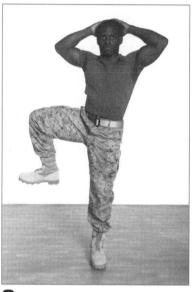

2 Lift your right knee and take it out to the side.

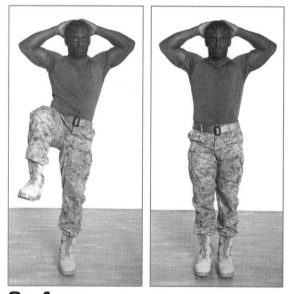

3–4 Rotate your right knee and hip forward through a full range of motion and step down.

Alternate legs.

To reverse direction, bring your right knee up in front of you and then rotate your right knee and hip to the side and back before stepping down.

Alternate legs.

★ SKIP & CLAP UNDER

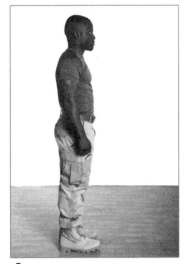

1 Stand upright.

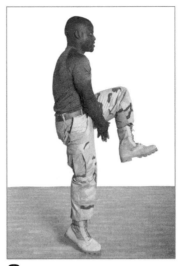

2 Starting with your left leg, skip forward, lifting your knee high enough to clap under your leg without allowing your chest to lean forward.

Alternate legs.

★ ANKLE TAP

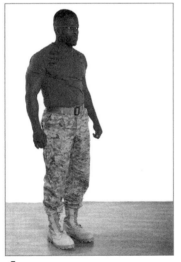

1 Stand upright.

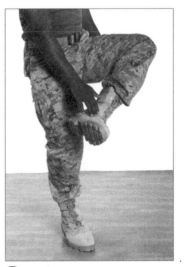

2 Starting with your left leg, skip forward, lifting your knee high enough to tap the inside of your ankle without allowing your chest to lean forward.

Alternate legs.

★ HIGH KNEES FORWARD & BACKWARD

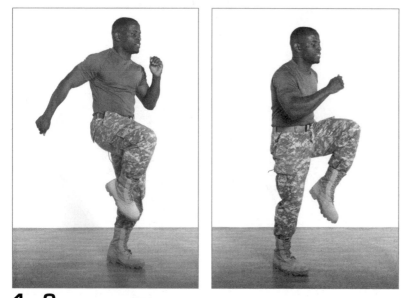

1–2 Jog forward while maintaining proper sprinting technique: Lean slightly forward, keep your arms bent 90 degrees and your shin slightly angled toward the ground. Drive your knees as high as possible, fully extend your push-off leg, and strike the ground with only the balls of your feet.

Once you've reached the set distance, perform the same drill moving backward.

★ HIGH KNEES IN PLACE

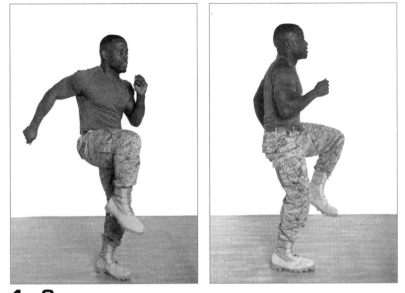

1-2 Moving in place, drive your knees as high as possible and quickly pump your arms. Your arms and legs should move in an alternating fashion.

★ LEG SWING FORWARD

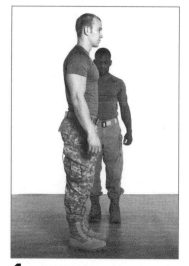

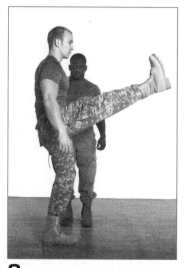

1 Stand upright. Place your hand on a tree, pole, wall or any other barrier for support if necessary.

2 Swing your leg forward, not allowing your foot to contact the ground.

Repeat and then switch legs.

★ LEG SWING ACROSS

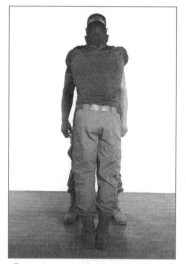

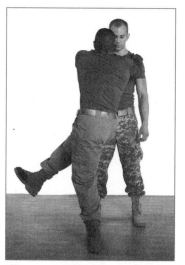

1 Stand upright with your hand(s) on a tree, pole, wall or any other barrier for support.

2 Swing your leg across your body, not allowing your foot to contact the ground.

Repeat and then switch legs.

★ 3 TO 9

This drill can be done in place or while moving forward.

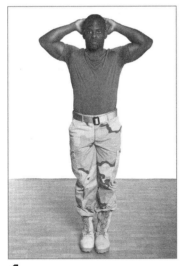

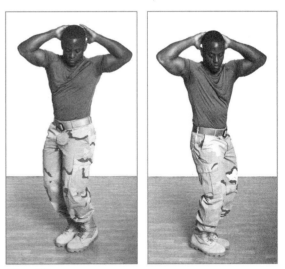

1 Stand upright with your hands placed on top of your head.

2–3 While bouncing continuously on the balls of your feet, quickly rotate your hips to the 3 o'clock and 9 o'clock positions.

★ ARM CIRCLE

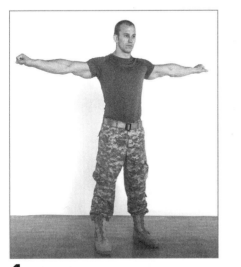

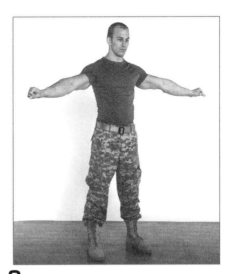

1 Stand upright with your arms extended out to the sides.

2 Rotate your arms forward in small circles, progressing to bigger circles.

Repeat the same motion moving backward.

★ ROLL-AROUND

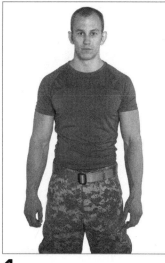

1 Stand upright.

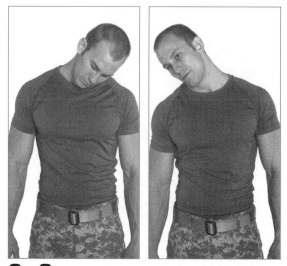

2–3 Roll your neck in a circular motion, first clockwise and then counterclockwise.

★ JACK IN A BOX

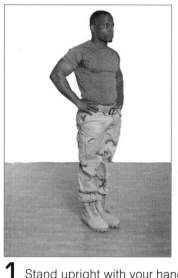

1 Stand upright with your hands on your hips.

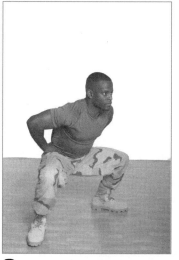

2 Drop into a squat position (toes pointed forward, back straight and thighs bent 90 degrees) and then quickly return to the start position.

★ CROSS-UP

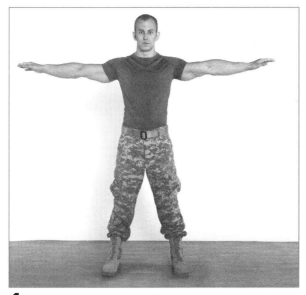

1 Stand upright with your feet and arms apart.

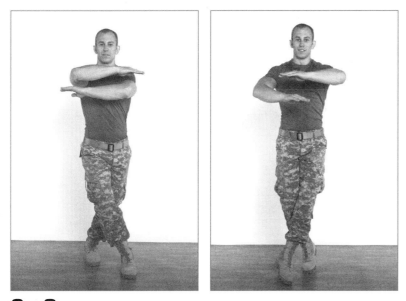

2–3 While bouncing continuously on the balls of your feet, simultaneously cross your arms and feet in an overlapping motion. Switch your feet and arms from top to bottom.

★ SHUFFLE & OVERHEAD ARM SWING

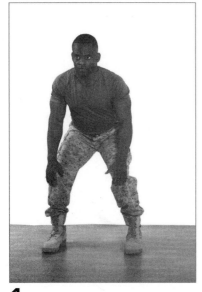

1 Assume an athletic position.

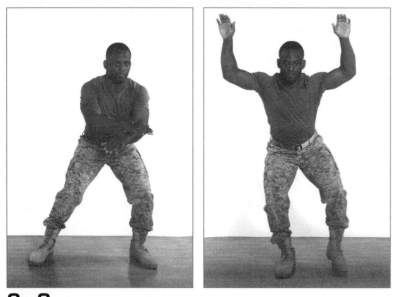

2-3 Shuffle laterally to your destination while simultaneously swinging your arms above your head.

Once you've reached your destination, return to starting position, repeating the same movement.

★ IN & OUT

Perform this drill as quickly as possible.

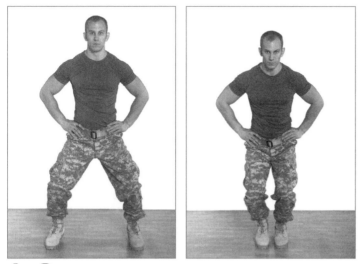

1-2 While standing upright with your hands on your hips, continuously bounce on the balls of your feet, bringing your feet in and out, as if doing jumping jacks without using your arms.

★ HEEL DIG & REACH

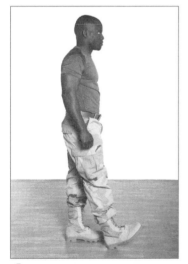 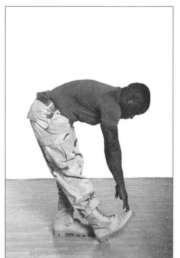

1 Stand upright and drive your right heel into the ground with your toe pointed upward.

2 Bend over and touch the top of your toe with both hands.

Switch sides.

★ WISHBONE

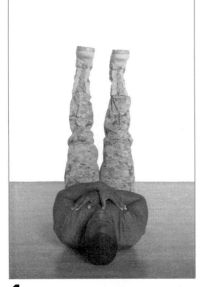

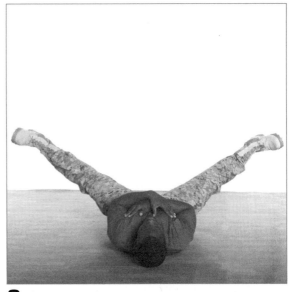

1 Lie on your back and cross your arms across your chest. Extend your legs with your heels pointed toward the sky.

2 Keeping your legs straight, continuously move your legs out to the sides and then back to starting position.

★ KICK-UP

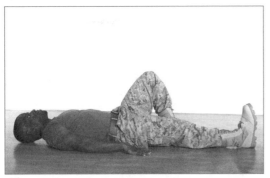

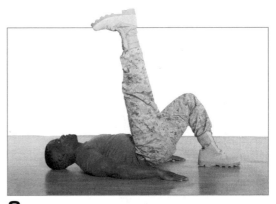

1 Lie on your back with your left leg bent with your foot on the ground and your right leg extended along the ground.

2 Kick your right leg toward your head.

Return to starting position. Repeat and then switch legs.

★ BALANCE & STABILITY ★ DRILLS

This section is designed to improve balance and stability in the lower extremities. Improving stability and balance increases overall physical performance and decreases the likelihood of lower extremity injuries.

★ SINGLE-LEG TOE TOUCH

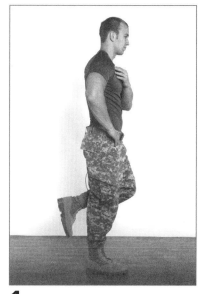

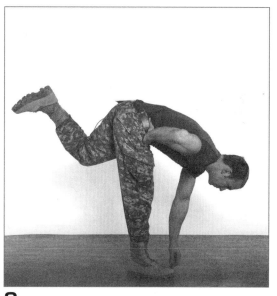

1 Stand on your right leg with your left leg bent roughly 90 degrees. Place your right hand on your waist and reach your left hand across your chest.

2 While maintaining your balance, bend at the hip and touch the top of your right foot with your left hand.

Return to starting position. Repeat and then switch legs.

★ STATUE OF LIBERTY

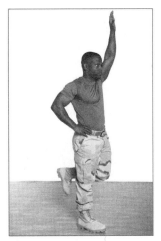

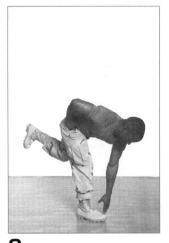

1 Stand on your right leg with your left leg bent roughly 90 degrees. Place your right hand on your waist and raise your left hand to the ceiling.

2 While maintaining your balance, bend at the hip and touch the top of your right foot with your left hand.

Return to starting position. Repeat and then switch legs.

★ REACH & PULL

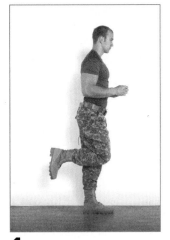

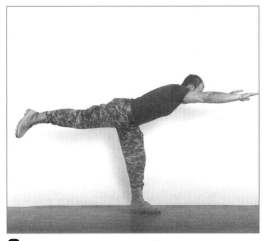

1 Stand on your left leg with your right leg and arms bent 90 degrees.

2 Slowly lean forward, extending your right leg backward and arms forward until your chest is parallel to the ground.

Return to starting position. Repeat and then switch legs.

★ REACH & HOLD

Unlike the Reach & Pull (page 56), this is a static hold instead of a dynamic movement.

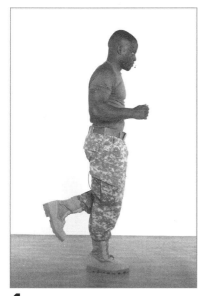

1 Stand on your right leg with your left leg and arms bent roughly 90 degrees.

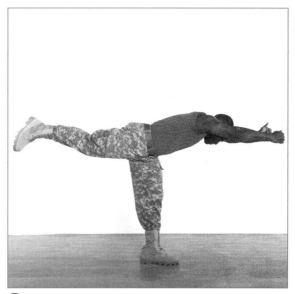

2 Slowly lean forward, extending your left leg and both arms until your chest is parallel to the ground. Hold this position for the exercise duration.

Return to starting position and repeat on your opposite side.

★ AROUND THE CLOCK

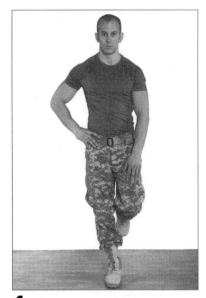

1 Stand on your right leg with your left leg bent 90 degrees; your lifted leg should never contact the ground. Place your right hand on your hip and left hand on your thigh.

2 With your left hand, reach for the 12 o'clock position (top of the toe) on your right foot.

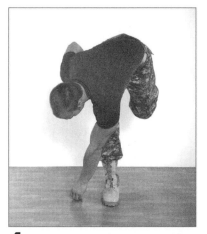

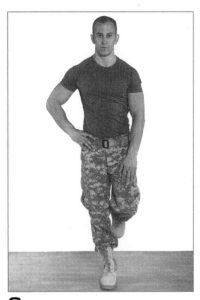

3 Return to starting position.

4 With your left hand, repeat the same movement for the 3 o'clock (inside of the foot), 6 o'clock (the heel) and 9 o'clock (outside of the foot) positions as well.

Repeat and then switch legs.

★ SINGLE-LEG HOP

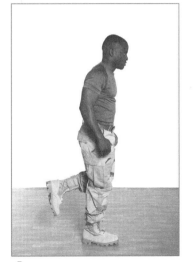 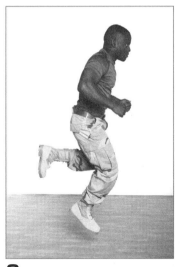

1 Stand on your right leg with your left leg bent roughly 90 degrees.

2 Hop forward to your destination, not allowing your opposite leg to contact the ground.

Return to starting position and switch sides.

★ SINGLE-LEG BACKWARD HOP

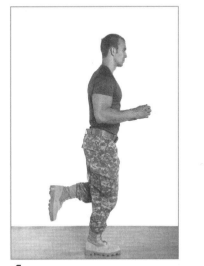 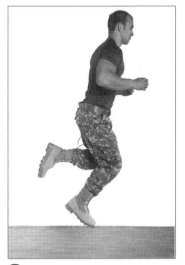

1 Stand on your right leg with your left leg bent 90 degrees.

2 Hop backward to your destination, not allowing your flexed leg to contact the ground.

Return to starting position and switch legs.

★ 3 HOPS & REACH

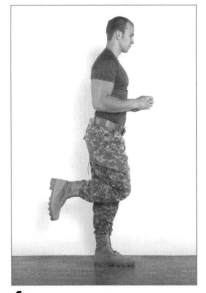

1 Stand on your left leg with your right leg and arms bent 90 degrees.

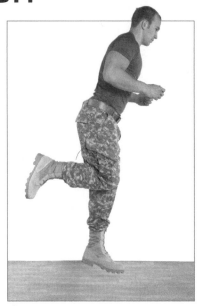

2 Hop forward 3 times.

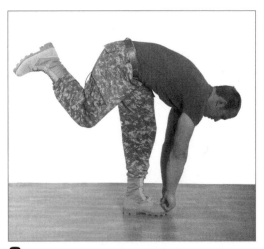

3 Bend at the hip and touch the top of your left toe with both hands.

Return to starting position. Repeat and then switch legs.

★ LATERAL HOP

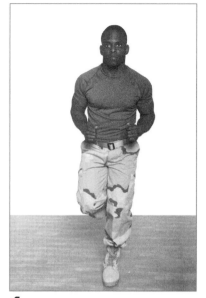

1 Stand on your left leg with your right leg bent 90 degrees.

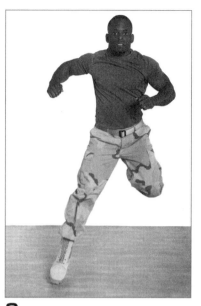

2 Laterally push off your left foot and land on your right foot.

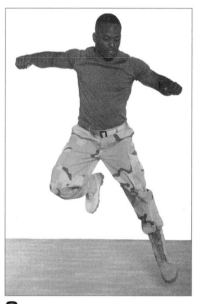

3 Now hop back to your left foot.

★ SINGLE-LEG 180

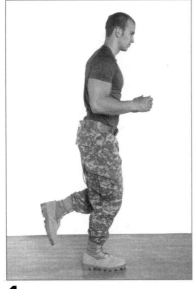

1 Stand on one foot.

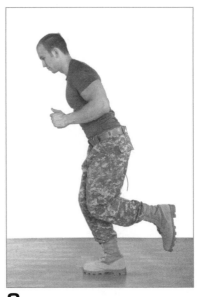

2 Jump 180 degrees, landing on the same leg. Maintain a slight bend in the knee to absorb the impact.

Repeat and then switch legs.

★ CORE EXERCISES ★

This section is designed to strengthen the core (abs). Strengthening your core will allow you to become a more functional athlete.

★ HELMET OBLIQUE TWIST

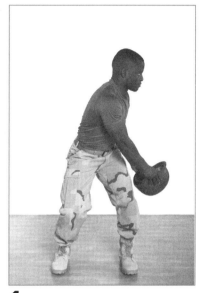

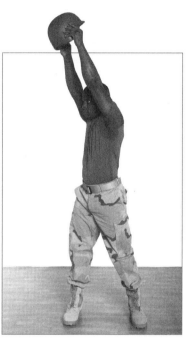

1 Stand with a slight bend in your knees and your helmet placed on the outside of your hip.

2 Rotate your torso upward and simultaneously bring your arms across your body in an upward diagonal angle until your arms and legs are extended.

Repeat and then switch sides.

★ CROSS-BODY CRUNCH

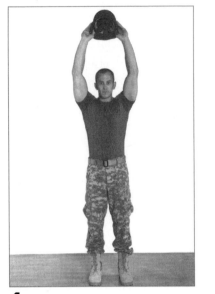

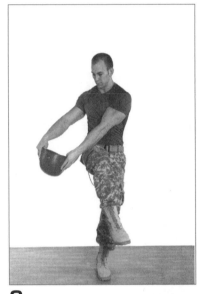

1 Stand upright with your helmet in your hands and your arms extended above your head.

2 Lower your arms in a downward diagonal angle toward your right while simultaneously lifting your right knee.

Alternate legs.

★ OVERHEAD KNEE TUCK

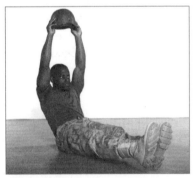

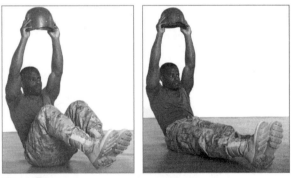

1 Sit on the ground with your arms extended above your head and your legs straight along the ground. Raise your legs a few inches off the ground. Maintain a flexed core and keep your arms extended above your head at all times.

2–3 Pull your knees toward your chest and then extend your legs back out. Your heels should not contact the ground.

★ SHIN GRAB

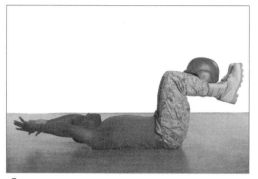

1 Lie on your back with your arms extended alongside your ears and your legs bent with your helmet placed on top of your shins. Maintain a flexed core at all times.

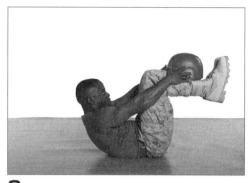

2 Bringing your shoulders off the ground, grab the helmet with both hands.

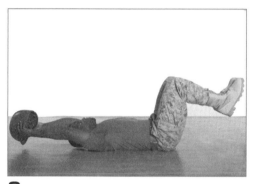

3 Extend both arms back alongside your ears.

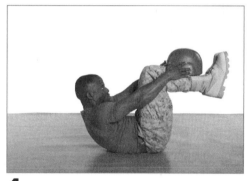

4 Touch the helmet to your shins.

Continue taking the helmet behind your head and to your shins. Each time you bring the helmet to your shins counts as one repetition.

★ CRUNCH EXTENSION

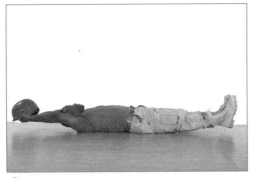

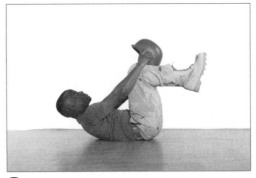

1 Lie on your back with your legs extended and your head and heels lifted 3 inches off the ground. Hold your helmet in both hands and extend your arms alongside your ears. Your head and heels should remain off the ground throughout the exercise.

2 While simultaneously bending your legs into a 90-degree angle, bring your arms forward and touch your shins with the helmet.

Return to starting position.

★ ALTERNATING V

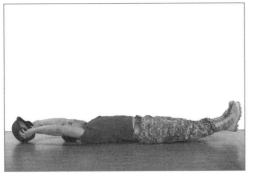

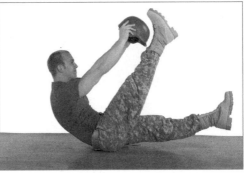

1 Lie on your back with your helmet in your hands and legs extended along the floor.

2 Simultaneously lift your upper body and right leg into a "V" shape, touching your shin with the helmet.

Lower to starting position and alternate legs.

★ ALTERNATING LEG EXTENSION

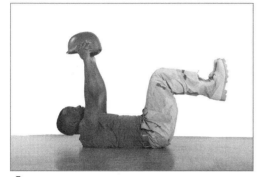 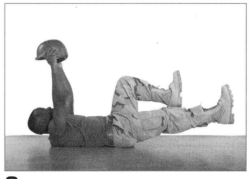

1 Lie on your back with your head lifted, arms extended up to the ceiling with your helmet in your hands, and legs bent 90 degrees. Your head and heels should stay off the ground throughout the exercise.

2 Maintaining the 90-degree angle with your right leg, extend your left leg, keeping it 3–5 inches off the ground. Hold this position for 3 seconds.

Alternate legs.

★ SEATED PUNCH

Perform this drill at a pace you can sustain for the exercise duration.

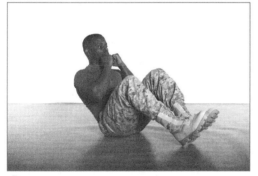 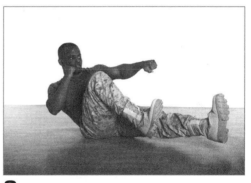

1 Sit on the ground with your knees slightly bent and heels lifted 3–5 inches. Maintain a straight back and flexed core for the duration of this exercise.

2 Punch with your left arm and simultaneously extend your left leg.

Upon full extension return to starting position. Continue alternating your legs and arms.

★ WEAVER

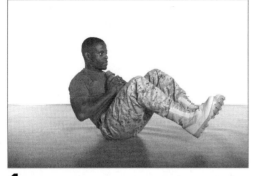

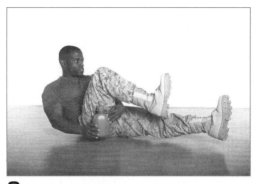

1 Sit on the ground with your heels lifted 3–5 inches off the ground, legs bent, core flexed and canteen held in both hands at approximately chest level. Your upper body is tilted slightly backward.

2 Extend one leg as you pull the opposite leg to your chest. Pass the canteen under the bent leg to the opposite hand.

Alternate sides.

★ HELMET TOSS & CATCH

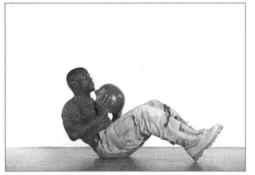

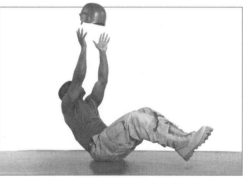

1 Sit on the ground with your heels lifted, back straight, knees bent and helmet in your hands at approximately chest level.

2 Keeping your legs bent and heels off the ground, toss the helmet above your head while maintaining a flexed core.

Catch and repeat.

★ HELMET TWIST

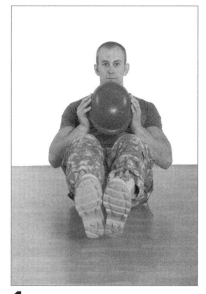

1 Sit on the ground with your heels lifted and helmet in your hands. Keep your back straight at all times during this exercise.

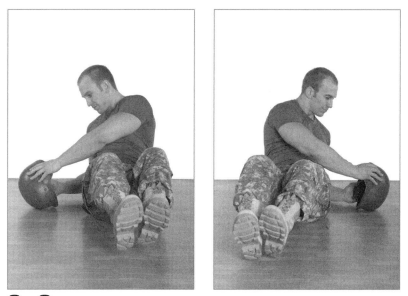

2-3 Twist your torso right to left as quickly as possible, touching the outside of your hip with your helmet.

★ HELMET TWIST & REACH

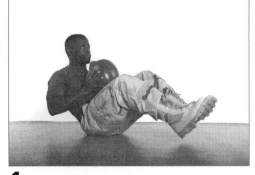

1 Sit on the ground with your heels lifted and helmet in your hands. Keep your back straight at all times during this exercise.

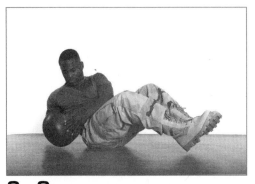

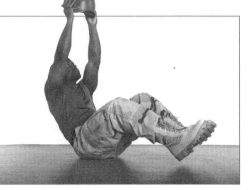

2-3 Twist your torso to the right and then reach for the sky.

Repeat to your left.

Continue alternating.

★ ELEVATED PLANK

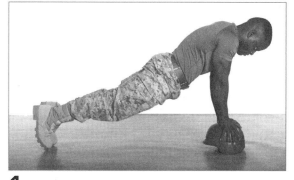

1 Place your helmet on the ground and both of your hands shoulder-width apart on top of the helmet. Assume the upward push-up position with your arms and legs fully extended. Your core and glutes should be flexed, and your hips shouldn't sag toward the ground. Maintain this position for the duration of the exercise.

★ DECLINE PLANK

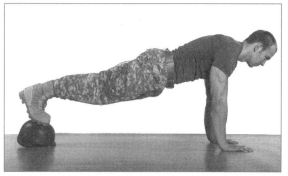

1 Place your helmet on the ground and both your feet on top of the helmet. Assume the upward push-up position with your hands shoulder-width apart on the ground and your arms and legs fully extended. Your core and glutes should be flexed, and your hips shouldn't sag toward the ground. Maintain this position for the duration of the exercise.

★ PLANK WITH KNEE TUCK

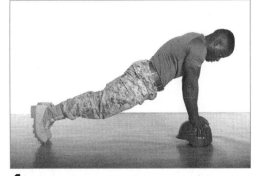

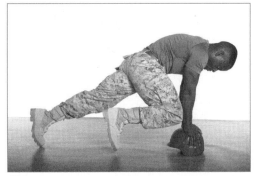

1 Place your helmet on the ground and your hands on top of the helmet. Assume plank position with your arms and legs fully extended.

2 Slide your right foot to the side and off the helmet and then bring your right knee to your right elbow.

Repeat to the other side and continue alternating.

★ HELMET PULL & TUCK

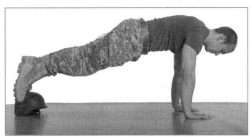

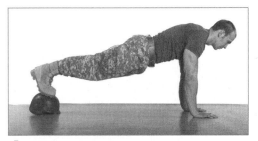

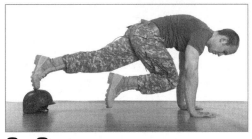

1 Unlike Plank with Knee Tuck, this is a three-part movement. Place your helmet on the ground and both your feet on top of the helmet. Assume the upward push-up position with your hands shoulder-width apart on the ground and your arms and legs fully extended.

2–3 Slide your right foot to the side and off the helmet and then bring your right knee toward your chest.

Return to starting position and switch sides.

★ PUSH-UP EXERCISES ★

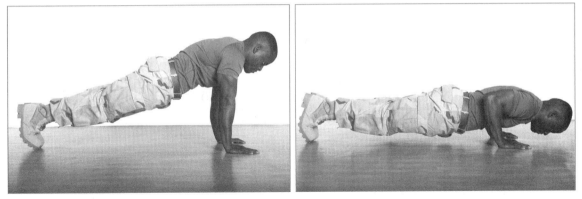

This section is designed to improve your upper-body strength with a variety of push-ups that offer a more challenging and exciting way to perform this traditional exercise. When performing a push-up, always keep your core tight and your body in good horizontal alignment, meaning your body should be in one straight horizontal line: Your butt shouldn't be too high or low, your hands should be approximately shoulder-width apart, your eyes are focused on the ground and your head is aligned with your shoulders. A good way to check your alignment is to place a book in the center of your back as you perform a push-up. If the book falls off, your body is not in a good horizontal alignment. If at any point the exercises are too challenging, you can modify them by starting from your knees.

★ HALF PUSH-UP

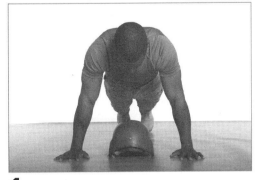

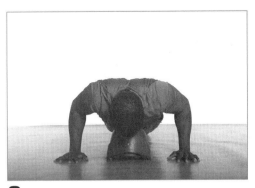

1 Start in the upward push-up position, with your chest centered directly over the helmet.

2 Lower yourself until your chest touches the helmet.

Return to starting position.

★ DECLINE HELMET PUSH-UP

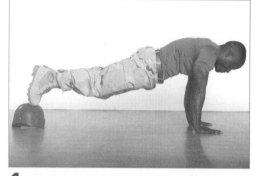

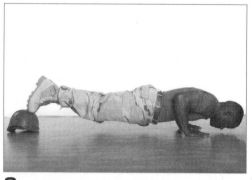

1 Place both feet on top of your helmet and assume the upward push-up position.

2 Lower down for the push-up.

Return to starting position.

★ CLOSE-GRIP CANTEEN PUSH-UP

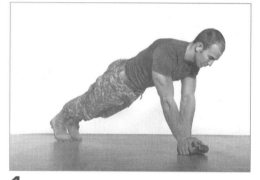

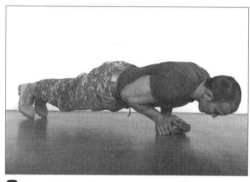

1 Place both hands on top of your canteen and assume the upward push-up position.

2 Lower down until your chest touches the canteen.

Return to starting position.

★ OFFSET-HAND PUSH-UP

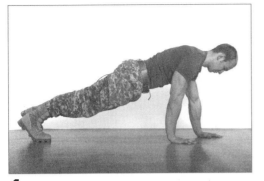 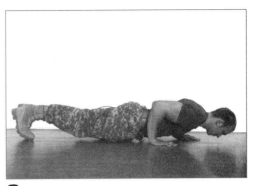

1 Start in the upward push-up position, with one of your hands positioned slightly forward of the other hand.

2 Lower your body until your arms reach a 90-degree angle.

Return to starting position and alternate hands.

★ CROSSOVER PUSH-UP

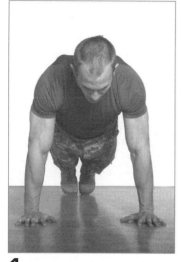

1 Start in the upward push-up position.

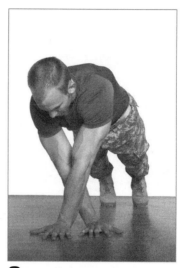

2 Cross your left hand over your right hand while moving to the right.

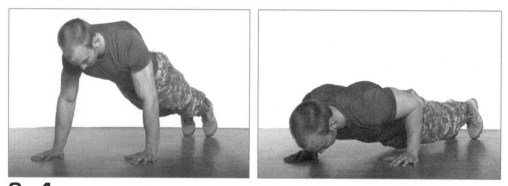

3–4 Uncross your hands by moving your right hand to the right and perform a push-up.

Repeat the same movement in the opposite direction.

★ HELMET 6-COUNT PUSH-UP

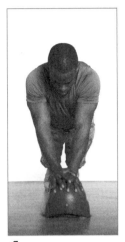

1 Place both hands on top of your helmet and assume the upward push-up position.

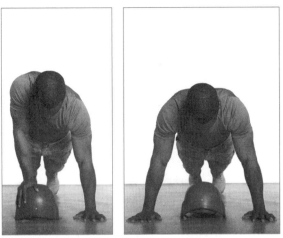

2–3 Keeping your arms fully extended, quickly place your left hand on the ground and then your right hand.

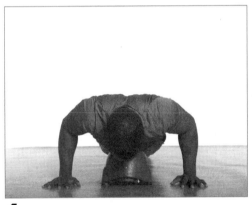

4 Now perform a push-up.

Quickly place your hands back on the helmet in the same order in which you removed them. Repeat this movement as quickly and accurately as possible.

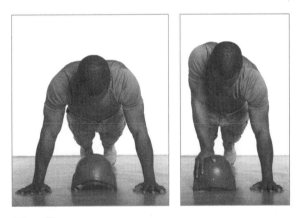

5–6 Quickly place your hands back on the helmet in the same order in which you removed them.

★ MOUNTAIN TOPPER

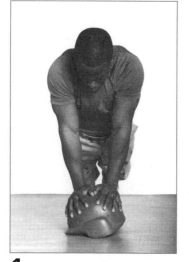

1 Place both hands on top of your helmet and assume the upward push-up position.

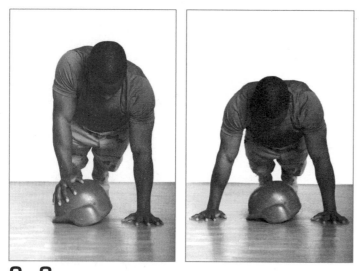

2–3 Keeping your arms fully extended, quickly take your left hand off the helmet, followed by your right hand, placing them on the floor to the side of the helmet.

Quickly replace your hands on the helmet in the order in which you removed them. Repeat this movement as quickly and accurately as possible.

★ ALTERNATING SHOULDER TAP PUSH-UP

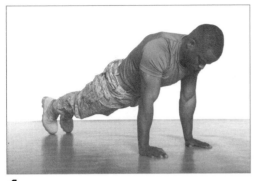

1 Start in the upward push-up position.

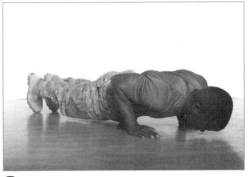

2 Lower down.

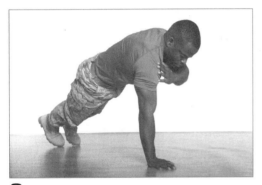

3 As you return to the upward position, tap your right shoulder with your left hand.

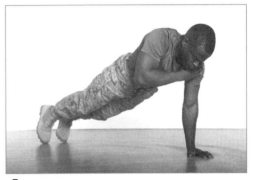

4 Now tap your left shoulder with your right hand.

★ PUSH-UP TO INCHWORM

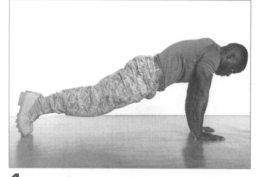

1 Start in the upward push-up position.

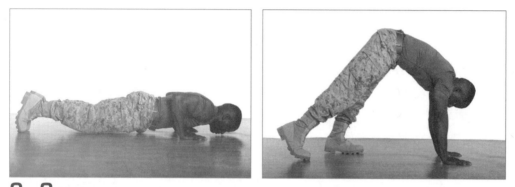

2–3 Perform a push-up and then slowly walk your feet toward your hands.

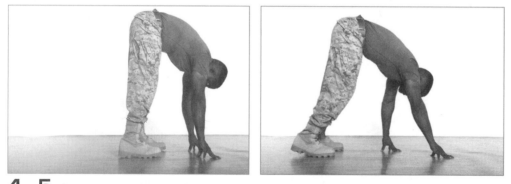

4–5 Once your feet have reached your hands or maximum flexibility level, walk your hands out until you're back in the upward push-up position.

★ KNEE TUCK PUSH-UP

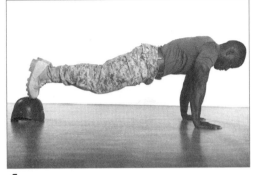

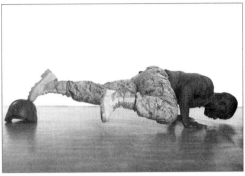

1 Place both feet on top of your helmet and assume the upward push-up position.

2 Lower down and simultaneously bring your right knee to your right elbow.

Return to starting position and alternate legs.

★ EXPLOSIVE PLYO PUSH-UP

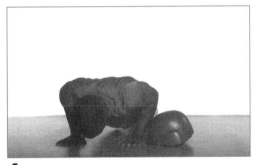

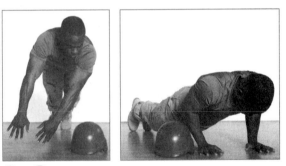

1 Start in the downward push-up position, with your helmet placed outside your left hand.

2–3 Explosively push your body in an upward lateral direction, landing on the opposite side of the helmet in the downward push-up position.

Reset and perform movement in the opposite direction.

★ HELMET PLYO PUSH-UP

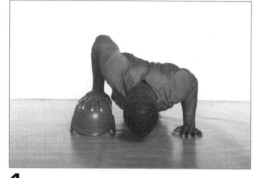

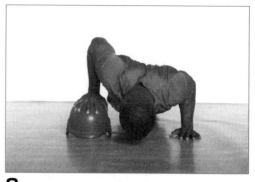

1 Start in the upward push-up position, with one hand on the helmet and your other hand on the ground.

2 Lower yourself until your chest touches the helmet.

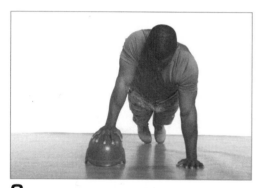

3 Explode up to starting position.

Repeat and then switch sides.

★ STRENGTH-TRAINING ★ EXERCISES

This section offers a variety of exercises utilizing your body weight, body armor and sandbags to improve your total-body strength.

★ BODY ARMOR BEAR CRAWL

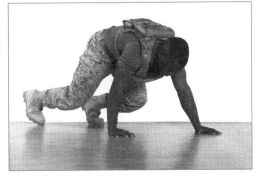 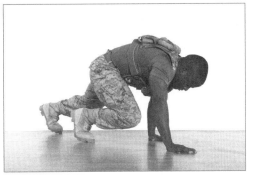

1–2 Start on your hands and toes with your knees off the ground, back straight, and butt low. Your hands and feet should remain shoulder-width apart and your knees should not contact the ground throughout the exercise. Moving forward, quickly bear crawl to your destination.

★ LATERAL CRAWL

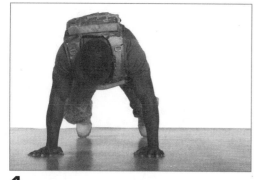

1 Start facedown on your hands and feet with your knees off the ground.

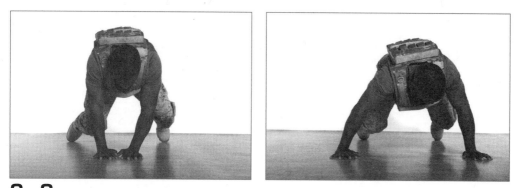

2–3 Without crossing your hands or feet, quickly bear crawl laterally to your destination. Your knees should not touch the ground.

Perform this drill in both directions.

★ BODY ARMOR CRAB WALK & KICK

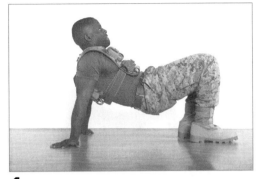

1 Sit on the ground with your hands on the ground behind you, feet on the floor and legs bent. Slightly raise your hips off the ground so that only your hands and feet are making contact with the ground.

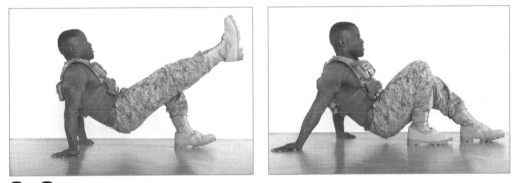

2−3 Crab walk backward by picking up one leg, kicking it straight and returning the same leg back to the ground.

Alternate leg kicks until you reach your destination.

★ MOUNTAIN CLIMBER

This is a stationary drill.

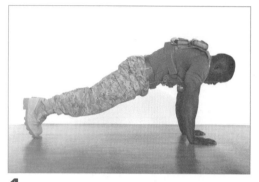

1 Start facedown on your hands and feet with your knees off the ground.

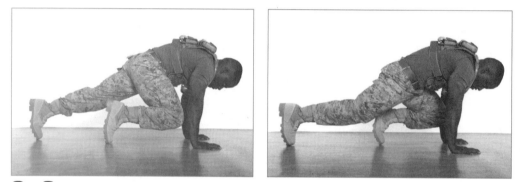

2–3 Quickly bring one knee to your chest, extend it back and then bring the other knee in.

Continue alternating.

★ DOUBLE TROUBLE

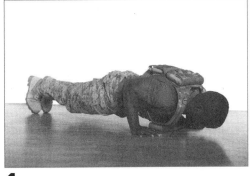

1 Start in the downward push-up position.

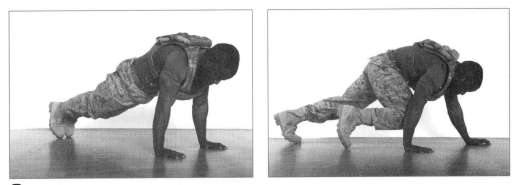

2 Perform 10 push-ups then bear crawl forward to your destination.

Once you've reached your destination, perform another 10 push-ups and then bear crawl backward to starting position.

★ THE BELASCO

Perform this drill as quickly as possible. Exercise distance can be longer or shorter than 10 yards.

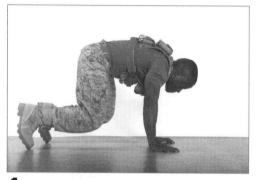

1 Start facedown on your hands and feet with your knees off the ground. Your knees shouldn't touch the ground throughout the exercise.

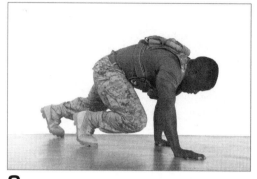

2 Bear crawl forward 10 yards.

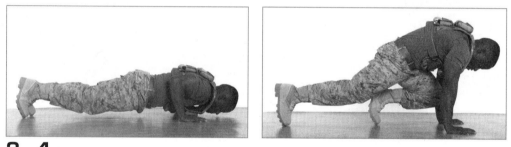

3–4 Immediately perform 10 push-ups and 10 mountain climbers.

Bear crawl forward another 10 yards and repeat 10 push-ups and 10 mountain climbers.

★ BENT-OVER ROW

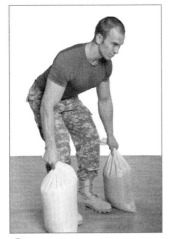

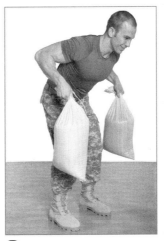

1 Start in a bent-over position, keeping your feet slightly apart, back flat, arms extended with a sandbag in each hand, chest parallel to the ground and knees slightly bent.

2 With your elbows against your rib cage, pull the sandbags up to your ribs and squeeze your back muscles. Slowly return to starting position.

★ ALTERNATING UPRIGHT ROW

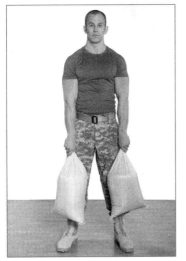

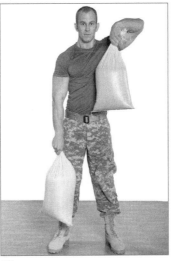

1 Stand with your feet shoulder-width apart and a sandbag in each hand.

2 With your left arm, perform an upright row by pointing your elbow up to the sky and bringing your hand to chin height.

Return to starting position. Alternate arms.

★ SHRUG TO UPRIGHT ROW

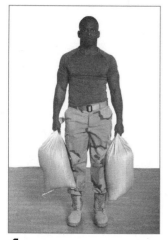

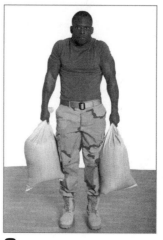

1 Stand with your feet shoulder-width apart and hold a sandbag in each hand.

2 Perform a shrug with both shoulders.

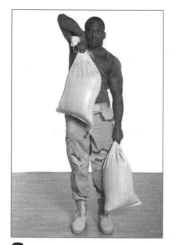

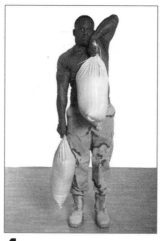

3 With your right arm, perform an upright row by pointing your elbow up to the sky and bringing your hand to your chin.

4 Return to starting position, perform a shrug with both shoulders and then perform an upright row with your left arm.

Continue alternating.

★ ROW

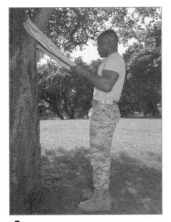

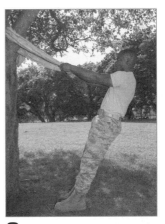

1 Loop a band around a sturdy tree, a pole or the sturdy loop of a truck, tank or Humvee and grab an end in each hand. Stand with your feet together, legs straight, and arms at a 90-degree angle and placed against your ribs.

2 Keeping your legs straight, slowly lower yourself downward and extend your arms. Make sure you don't bend at the waist during the downward phase.

Once your arms have reached full extension, pull your body upward to the start position.

★ SINGLE-ARM PULL

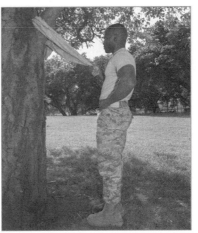

1 Loop a band around a sturdy tree, a pole or the sturdy loop of a truck, tank or Humvee and grab both ends in one hand. Stand with your feet together and legs straight. Your body is positioned with a backward tilt and your pulling arm is fully extended. Place your non-pulling hand on your hip.

2 Slowly pull your body into the upright position or until you've reached maximum range of motion.

Slowly return to starting position. Repeat and then switch sides.

★ PULL-APART

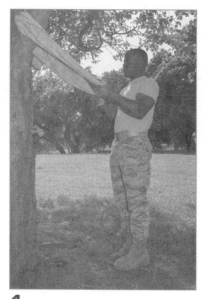

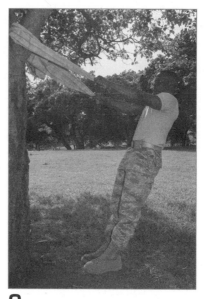

1 Loop a band around a sturdy tree, a pole or the sturdy loop of a truck, tank or Humvee and grab an end in each hand. Stand with your feet together and arms at a 90-degree angle and placed against your ribs.

2 Keeping your legs straight, slowly lower yourself into a downward tilt position until your arms reach full extension. Make sure you don't bend at the waist during the downward phase and only utilize the muscles of the upper body.

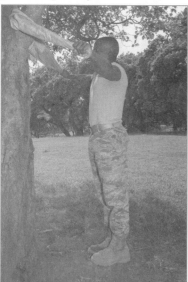

3 Return to the upward position and simultaneously open your arms to the sides in the formation of a "T."

★ OVERHEAD SANDBAG PRESS

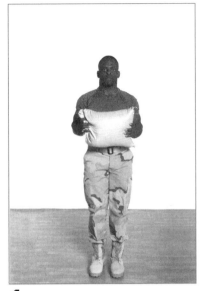

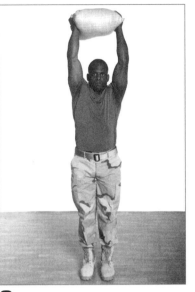

1 Stand with your feet shoulder-width apart and hold a sandbag against your chest.

2 Press the sandbag over your head until your arms are fully extended.

Return to starting position.

★ SANDBAG CHEST PRESS

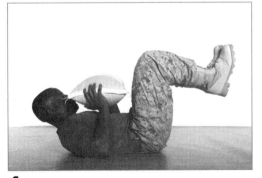

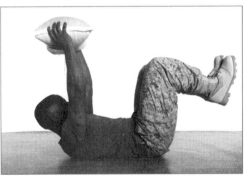

1 Lie on your back with your legs bent 90 degrees and hold a sandbag in both hands approximately 3–5 inches from your chest. Lift your head and focus your eyes on your thighs.

2 Press the sandbag upward until your arms are fully extended.

Return to starting position.

★ SANDBAG CHEST PRESS & LEG EXTENSION

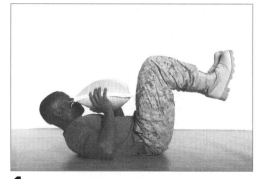

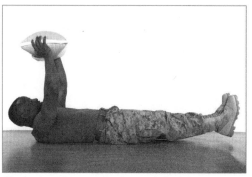

1 Lie on your back with your legs bent 90 degrees and hold a sandbag in both hands approximately 3–5 inches from your chest. Lift your head and focus your eyes on your thighs.

2 Simultaneously press the sandbag upward and extend your legs forward.

Return to starting position.

★ SANDBAG BICEPS CURL

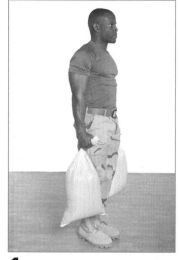

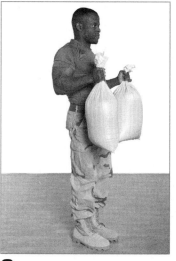

1 Stand with your feet shoulder-width apart and hold a sandbag in each hand.

2 Curl the sandbags upward until you've reached maximum range of motion or the tops of your shoulders.

Return to starting position. Alternate arms.

★ SINGLE-ARM ISOLATION HOLD

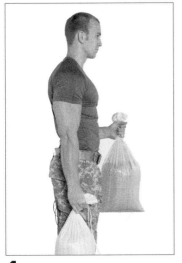

1 Stand with a sandbag in each hand and one arm positioned by your waist at a 90-degree angle. Maintain this position for the duration of the exercise. Alternate arms.

★ SANDBAG CARRY

Perform as many laps as possible for the duration of the exercise. Down and back is 1 lap.

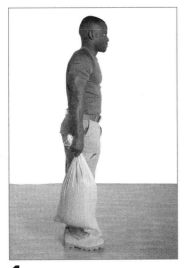

1 Stand with a sandbag in each hand

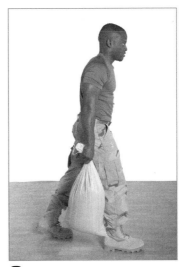

2 Quickly walk (don't run) to your destination.

★ SANDBAG SWING

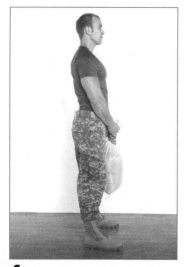

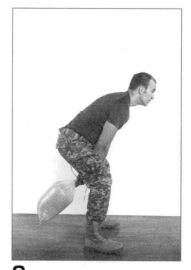

1 Stand with your feet shoulder-width apart and arms straight, holding a sandbag in both hands. Your arms should remain straight during this exercise.

2 To generate momentum, slowly push back your hips and tilt your upper body forward, causing the sandbag to swing between your legs.

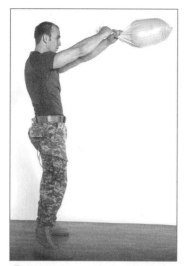

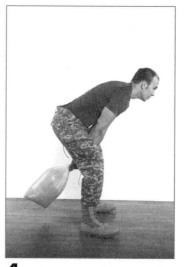

3 Once your arms have reached maximum range of motion, quickly thrust your hips forward and squeeze your butt cheeks until your body reaches a vertical position, causing the sandbag to swing in an upward motion, approximately shoulder to eye level.

4 Allow the sandbag to follow the same path down between your legs, continuing to use your hips to maintain the swing.

★ SINGLE-ARM SANDBAG SWING

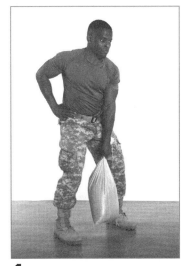

1 Stand with your feet shoulder-width apart, with one hand placed on your waist and the other arm extended and holding the sandbag. Your swinging arm should remain straight during this exercise.

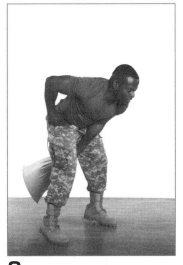

2 To generate momentum, slowly push back your hips and tilt your upper body forward, causing the sandbag to swing between your legs.

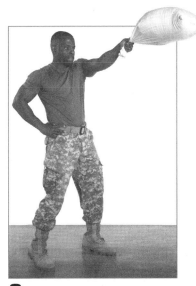

3 Once your arm has reached maximum range of motion, quickly thrust your hips forward, causing the sandbag to swing in an upward motion, approximately shoulder to eye level.

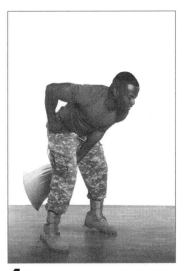

4 Allow the sandbag to follow the same path down between your legs, continuing to use your hips to maintain the swing.

★ ALTERNATING LUNGE

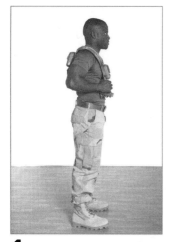

1 Stand with your feet shoulder-width apart.

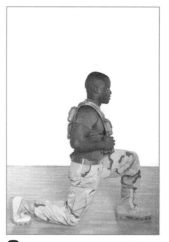

2 Step forward with your left leg until both knees reach 90 degrees. Your back knee should not contact the ground.

Return to starting position. Switch sides, and continue alternating.

★ STATIC LUNGE & OVERHEAD PRESS

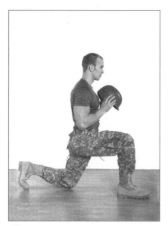

1 Assume the split lunge position, with both of your legs bent 90 degrees, your back knee off the ground, and your helmet held against your chest.

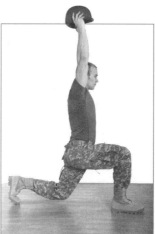

2 Press the helmet above your head, extending your arms fully.

Return to starting position. Switch leg position and repeat.

★ STATIC SPLIT LUNGE & FRONT PRESS

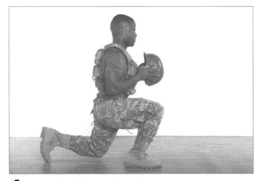

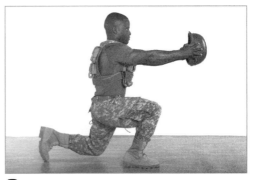

1 Assume the split lunge position, with both of your legs bent 90 degrees, your back knee off the ground, and your helmet held against your chest.

2 Press your helmet forward, extending your arms fully.

Return to starting position.

Switch leg position and repeat.

★ SQUAT

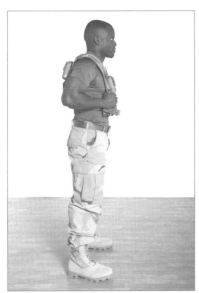

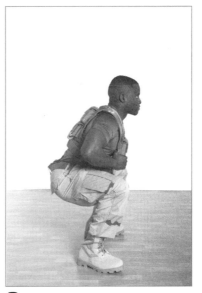

1 Stand with your feet shoulder-width apart and your hands against your chest.

2 Keeping your heels on the ground, slowly lower your butt until your thighs reach 90 degrees.

Return to starting position.

★ SQUAT TO PRESS

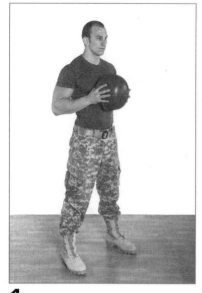

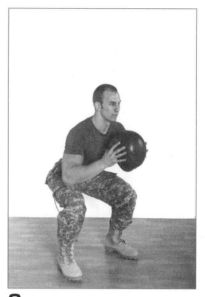

1 Stand with your feet shoulder-width apart and your helmet held against your chest.

2 Keeping your heels on the ground, slowly lower your butt until your thighs reach 90 degrees.

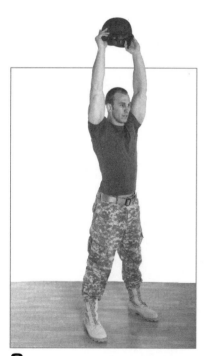

3 Return to starting position and simultaneously press the helmet above your head.

★ SINGLE-LEG SQUAT

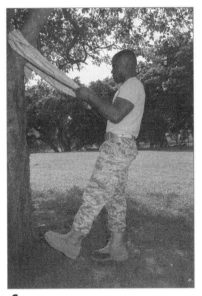
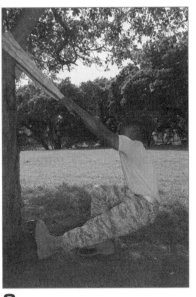

1 Loop a band around a sturdy tree, a pole or the sturdy loop of a truck, tank or Humvee and grab an end in each hand. Stand on your left leg with your right leg lifted 3–5 inches off the ground, your arms slightly bent and your elbows at your ribs.

2 Slowly lower yourself until your arms reach full downward extension and your left thigh reaches 90 degrees.

Return to starting position.

Repeat and then switch sides.

★ SANDBAG SQUAT & PRESS

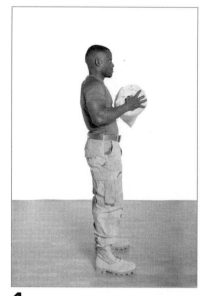

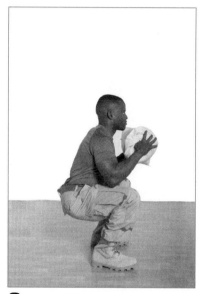

1 Stand with your feet shoulder-width apart and hold a sandbag against your chest.

2 Keeping your heels on the ground, slowly lower your butt until your thighs reach 90 degrees.

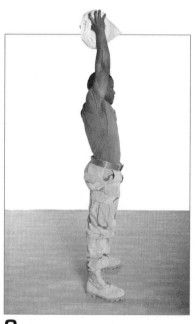

3 Return to starting position and simultaneously press the sandbag above your head.

★ PUSH TOSS

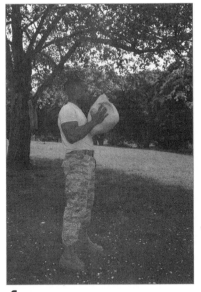

1 Stand with your feet shoulder-width apart and hold a sandbag against your chest.

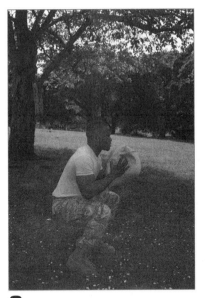

2 Keeping your heels on the ground, slowly lower your butt until your thighs reach 90 degrees.

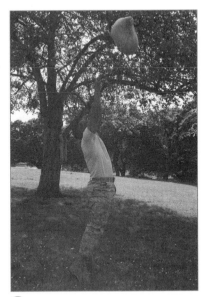

3 Quickly return to starting position and simultaneously release the sandbag upward at the end of the movement. Allow the sandbag to hit the ground upon release before performing the next repetition.

★ TWIST & TOSS

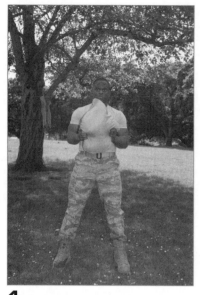

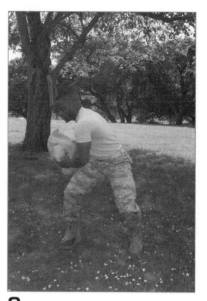

1 Stand with your feet shoulder-width apart and hold a sandbag with both hands against your chest.

2 Slowly twist downward, bringing the sandbag to the outside of one knee.

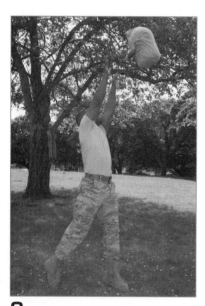

3 Quickly twist upward in the opposite direction and toss the sandbag upward.

Allow the sandbag to hit the ground upon release before performing the next repetition.

★ BACKWARD TOSS

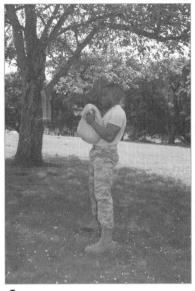

1 Stand with your feet shoulder-width apart and hold a sandbag with both hands against your chest.

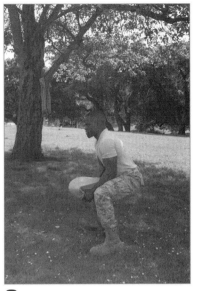

2 Keeping your heels on the ground, slowly lower your butt until your thighs reach 90 degrees.

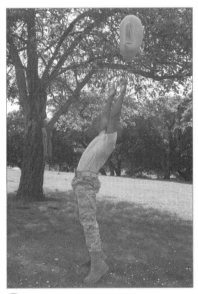

3 Quickly stand up and release the sandbag over your head when your body has reached full extension. Your upward motion should feel as if you were performing a fast upward squat.

Allow the sandbag to hit the ground upon release before performing the next repetition.

★ PUSH-UP TO SQUAT TOSS

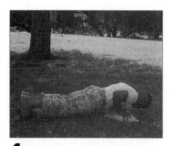

1 Assume a downward push-up position with both hands on the sandbag.

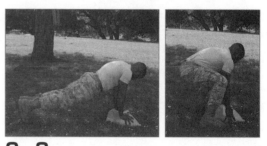

2–3 Perform a push-up then quickly jump your feet to the downward squat position. Grab the sandbag in both hands as you transition from the push-up into the downward squat.

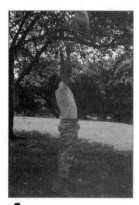

4 Quickly stand up and release the sandbag upward when your body has reached full extension.

Allow your sandbag to hit the ground upon release before performing the next repetition.

★ PARTNER EXERCISES ★

The following exercises are to be performed with a partner. Not only do you receive a great workout, so does your partner.

★ PARTNER PROGRESSION & STATIONARY SPRINT

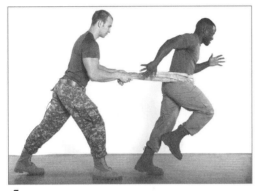

1 Sprint as quickly as possible to your destination while your partner applies resistance by holding a combat top tightly around your waist. Always maintain a slight forward lean, a roughly 90-degree bend in your arms and a parallel shin angle while driving your knees forward and striking the ground with the balls of your feet.

★ COMBAT UNIFORM SHUFFLE

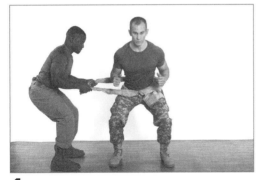

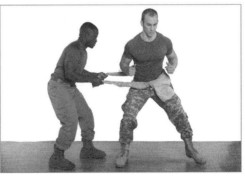

1 Start in the athletic position with your partner holding a combat uniform tightly around your waist.

2 Not allowing your body to turn or feet to cross, shuffle laterally to your destination as your partner applies resistance.

Perform the drill in both directions.

★ COMBAT UNIFORM SHUFFLE & TOUCH

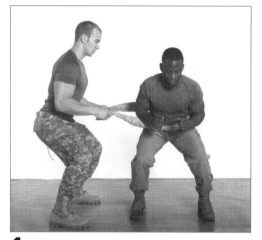

1 Start in the athletic position with your partner holding the combat uniform tightly around your waist.

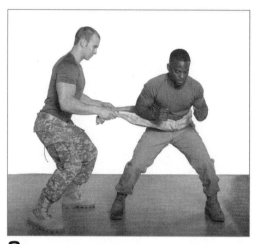

2 Not allowing your body to turn or feet to cross, shuffle laterally to your destination as your partner applies resistance.

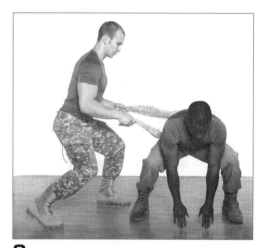

3 Once you reach your destination, drop your hips and touch the ground with both hands.

Perform the drill in both directions.

★ COMBAT UNIFORM BACKPEDAL

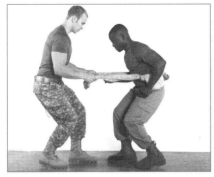

1 Stand facing your partner with your partner holding a combat uniform tightly around your waist. Now bend your knees 90 degrees and keep your chest up. Maintain this position for the duration of the exercise.

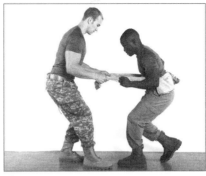

2 Not allowing your body to turn, quickly walk backward to your destination as your partner applies resistance. Down and back is 1 repetition.

★ RESISTANCE PUSH-UP

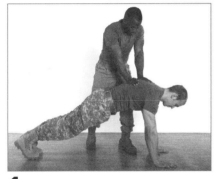

1 Assume an upward push-up position with your partner's hands placed in the middle of your back.

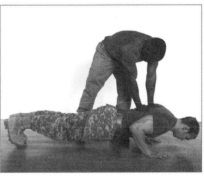

2 Perform a push-up as your partner applies continuous resistance. If your partner is applying too much resistance, he should remove one hand from your back.

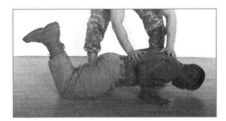

Modification: You can also perform the push-up from your knees.

★ WHEEL BARROW PUSH-UP

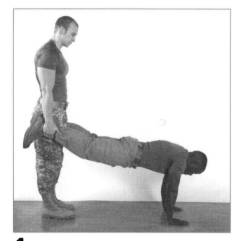

1 Assume the upward decline push-up position with your ankles placed in your partner's hands.

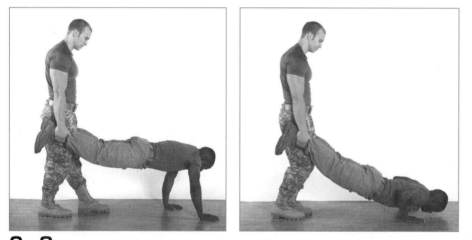

2–3 With your partner grasping your ankles, walk on your hands 10 steps then perform your desired number of push-ups, maintaining the decline position.

★ PARTNER PULL-UP

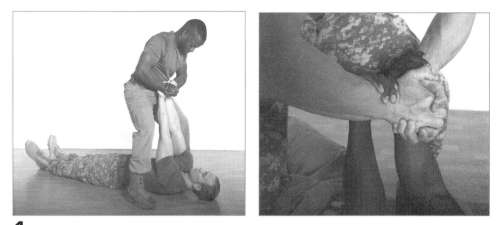

1 Lie on your back with your legs straight on the ground. Your partner should be straddled over your chest with a slight bend at the waist, hands together, feet apart, chest up and back straight. Extend your arms and grab your partner's forearms using an underhand grip.

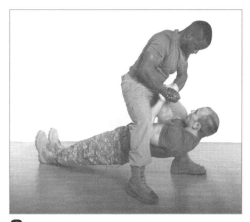

2 Slowly pull yourself up until your chest touches your partner's hands.

Return to starting position.

★ AROUND THE WORLD

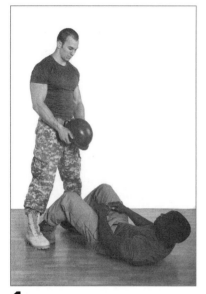

1 Lie on your back with your partner holding a helmet at the base of your feet.

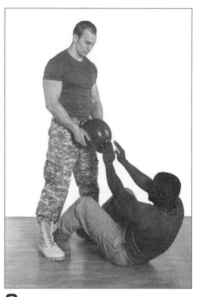

2 Perform a sit-up and touch the helmet when you're at the up position.

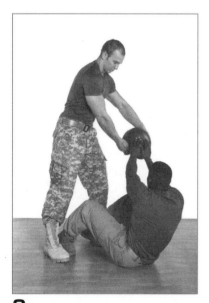

3 Return to starting position. Continue the sit-up with your partner moving the helmet to a variety of locations (left, right, up, down) for you to reach.

★ HELMET PRESS

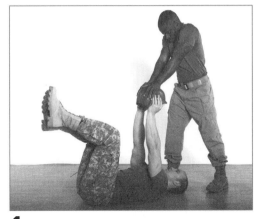

1 Lie on your back with your helmet in your hands, arms extended above your face and legs bent 90 degrees. Your partner should be standing over your head with arms fully extended, feet apart, chest up, back straight and hands placed on top of your helmet.

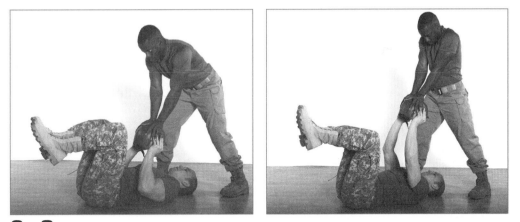

2–3 Move your helmet upward and downward as your partner applies continuous resistance.

★ SINGLE-LEG CURL

Your partner should continuously apply resistance during the upward and downward phases.

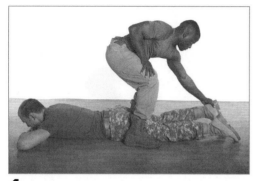

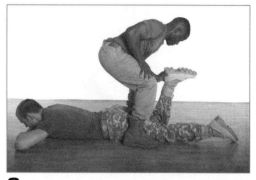

1 Lie facedown with your partner standing with his legs on either side of your butt, facing your feet. Your partner should have a slight bend at the waist, with his back straight and his left hand clutching the back of your right heel.

2 With your heel in your partner's hand, slowly pull your leg to a 90-degree angle.

Return to starting position. Repeat, then switch sides.

★ DOUBLE-LEG CURL

Your partner should continuously apply resistance during the upward and downward phases.

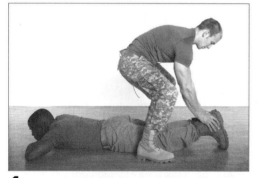

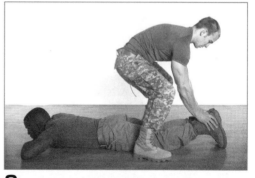

1 Lie facedown with your partner standing with his legs on either side of your butt, facing your feet. Your partner should have a slight bend at the waist, with back straight and hands clutching the backs of your heels.

2 With your heels in your partner's hand, slowly pull your legs to a 90-degree angle.

Return to starting position.

★ BUDDY CARRY

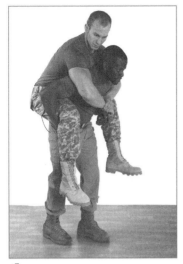

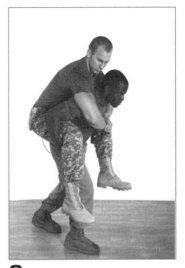

1 Begin with your partner straddled across your back. Your arms should be placed around your partner's legs and your partner's arms should be folded around your shoulders.

2 Carry your partner to your destination as quickly as possible. Down and back is 1 repetition.

★ NECK STRENGTHENING 1

This can be done with both partners standing or sitting.

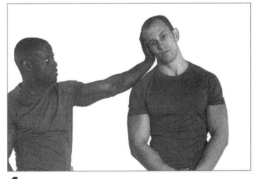

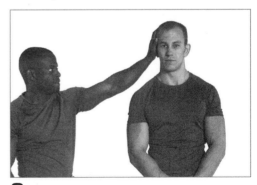

1 Maintaining a vertical alignment with your upper body, place your ear against your partner's hand. Your partner's arm should be completed extended.

2 Slowly move your head against your partner's hand as your partner applies resistance. All movement should come from your neck, not your shoulders.

Once your neck reaches maximum range of motion, return to starting position. Repeat and then switch sides.

★ NECK STRENGTHENING 2

This can be done with both partners standing or sitting.

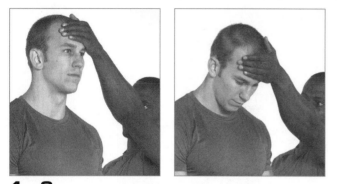

1-2 Maintaining a vertical alignment with your upper body, place your forehead against your partner's hand. Your partner's arm should be completely extended. Slowly move your head against your partner's hand as your partner applies resistance. All movement should come from your neck, not your shoulders.

Once your neck reaches maximum range of motion, return to starting position.

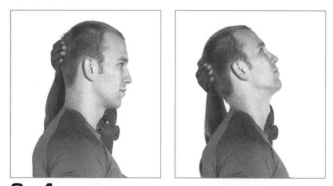

3-4 Now place the back of your head against your partner's hand. Slowly move your head against your partner's hand as your partner applies resistance.

Once your neck reaches maximum range of motion, return to starting position.

★ AGILITY, SPEED, ★ & PLYOMETRICS

The drills in this section have been designed to improve your lateral and linear speed, imitating movement patterns often utilized during military training. Perform these drills at maximum effort. Remember: Your focus is speed and accuracy.

Here are some positions you should familiarize yourself with before starting the drills.

HAND GRIP

Use one of these hand grips when performing the drills.

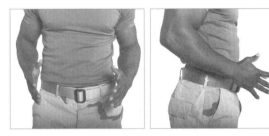
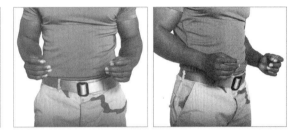

Open-Hand Grip: Your hands are completely open in a relaxed position.

Pinch Grip: Your index finger and thumb are lightly placed together.

ATHLETIC POSITION

This is your starting and finishing position for all jumping, shuffling and backpedaling exercises.

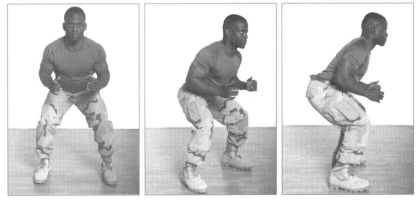

Stand with your feet shoulder-width apart, keeping a slight bend in your hips and knees, and arms bent by your sides.

★ ARM SWING (RUNNING FORM)

The purpose of this drill is to your improve upper-body running mechanics. During this drill you should move your arms as rapidly as possible while standing in place. Utilize this technique when performing running and backpedaling drills.

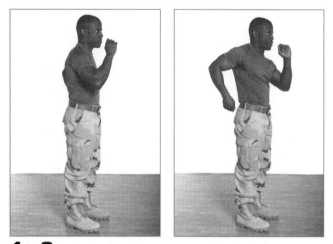

1–2 Your arms are at 90 degrees and your arm movement should occur from your shoulders. Quickly pump your arms from your chin to your hip, not allowing your arms to cross your body.

★ STATIONARY FEET SWITCH

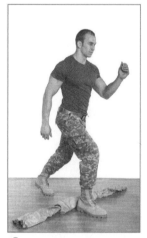

1 Start with each foot on opposite sides of a combat uniform.

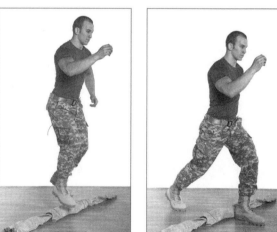

2–3 Jump slightly off the ground and switch your foot position mid-air, striking the ground with only the balls of your feet. Perform this drill as quickly as possible.

★ LATERAL HOP

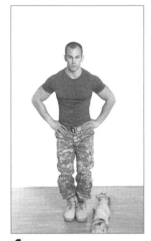

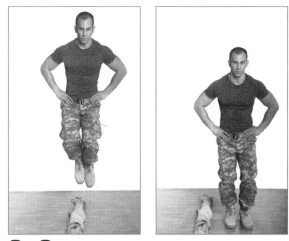

1 Stand to the right of a combat uniform and place your hands on your hips, keeping your knees slightly bent.

2–3 Quickly hop from side to side over the uniform, striking the ground with only the balls of your feet.

★ QUICK SPRINT

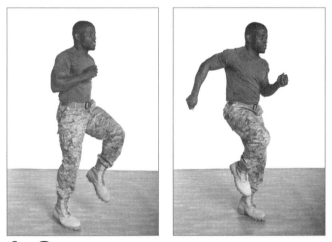

1–2 Sprint in place as quickly as possible, fully extending your push-off leg. Always maintain a slight forward lean, a 90-degree bend in your arms and a parallel shin angle while striking the ground with the balls of your feet.

★ SQUAT JUMP

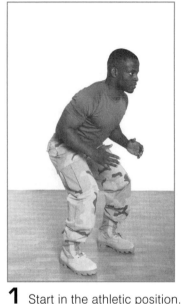

1 Start in the athletic position.

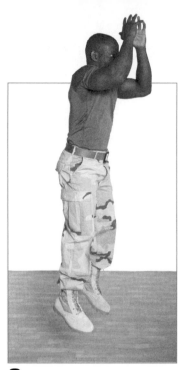

2 Rapidly move your arms upward and explosively jump.

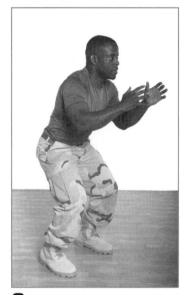

3 Absorb the impact of the landing by maintaining a slight bend in your knees.

★ LATERAL QUICK SHUFFLE

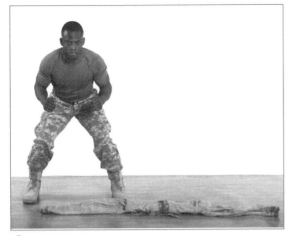

1 Start in the athletic position.

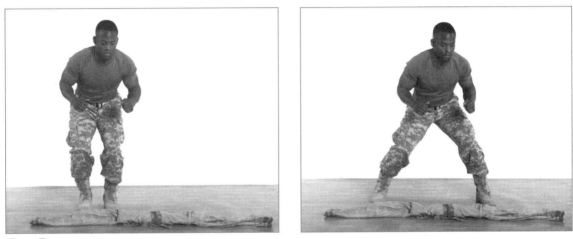

2-3 Quickly shuffle laterally to the opposite end of your combat uniform.

Quickly return to starting position.

★ SHUFFLE & TOUCH

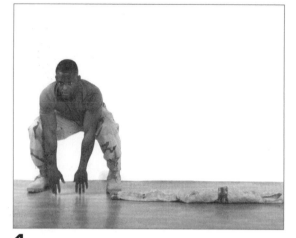

1 Start in the athletic position with all of your fingertips touching the ground.

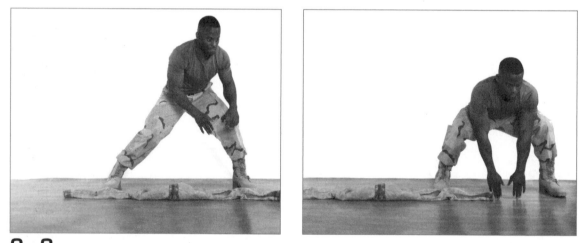

2–3 Quickly shuffle laterally to the opposite end of your combat uniform, touch the ground and then quickly return to starting position.

★ STATIONARY TOP TO BOTTOM

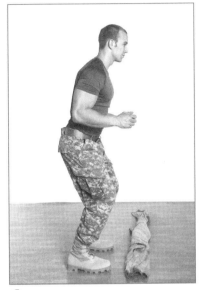

1 Start in the athletic position at one end of your combat uniform.

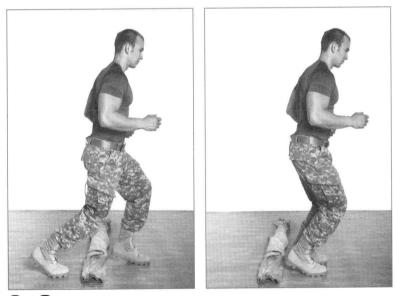

2-3 Striking the ground with only the balls of your feet, step to the opposite side of your combat uniform, leading with your left foot, followed by your right foot.

Use the same foot pattern when you return to starting position.

★ PUSH-UP TO SHUFFLE

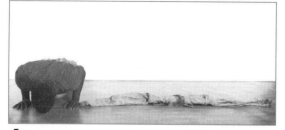

1 Assume the downward push-up position.

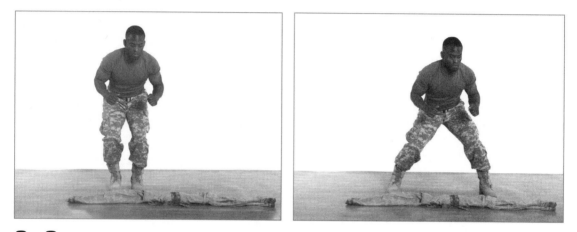

2-3 Perform 1 push-up, jump to your feet and quickly shuffle to the opposite end of your combat uniform.

Once you reach the opposite end, perform another push-up and then quickly shuffle to starting position.

★ QUICK SHUFFLE & JUMP

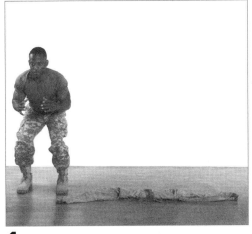

1 Start in the athletic position.

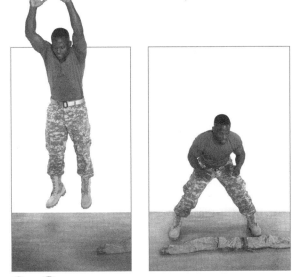

2–3 Perform 1 squat jump and then quickly shuffle to the opposite end of your combat uniform.

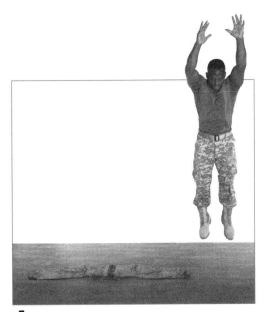

4 Once you reach the opposite end, perform another squat jump and then quickly shuffle to starting position.

★ SPRINT TO BACKPEDAL

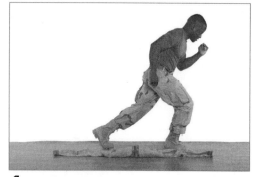

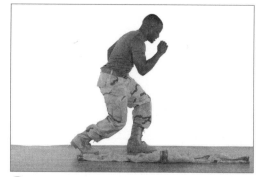

1 Sprint to the opposite end of your combat uniform.

2 Once you reach the end, drop your hips and backpedal to starting position.

★ HELMET TOE TAP

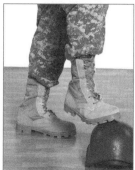

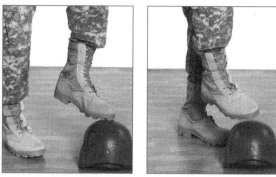

1 Stand with your right foot on top of your helmet and your left foot on the ground.

2–3 Bouncing on the balls of your feet, continuously switch your foot position, touching the top of the helmet with your toes each repetition.

★ 360° SHUFFLE

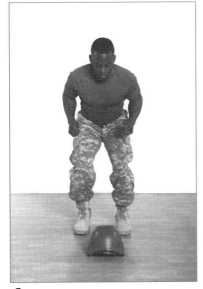

1 Start in the athletic position with your helmet on the ground in front of your feet.

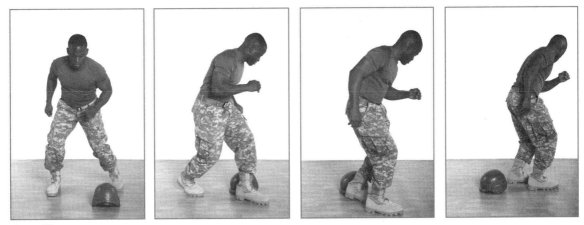

2–5 Without crossing your feet, make a 360-degree shuffle around the helmet.

Repeat this drill in the opposite direction.

★ HELMET JUMPOVER

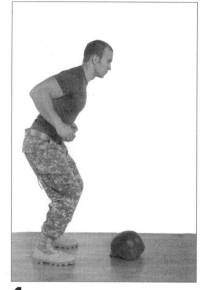

1 Start in the athletic position with your helmet on the ground in front of your feet.

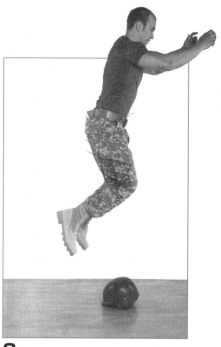

2 Rapidly move your arms upward and explosively jump over the helmet.

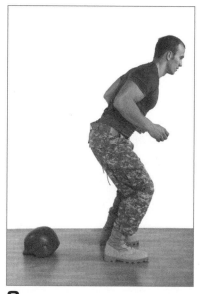

3 Absorb the impact of the landing by maintaining a slight bend in your knees.

★ HELMET JUMPOVER & TURN

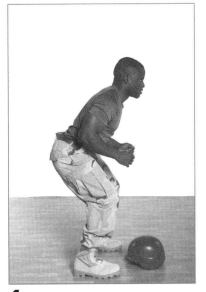

1 Start in the athletic position with your helmet on the ground in front of your feet.

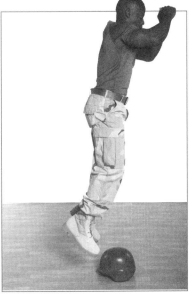

2 Rapidly move your arms upward and explosively jump over the helmet.

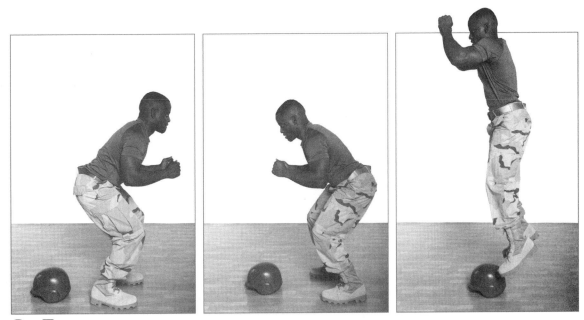

3–5 Upon landing, make a quick jump-turn to face the helmet and then jump over the helmet again.

Perform this drill as quickly as possible.

★ 4 TOE TAPS TO 360° SHUFFLE

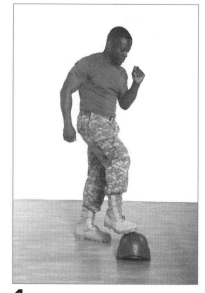

1 Stand with your right foot on your helmet and your left foot on the ground.

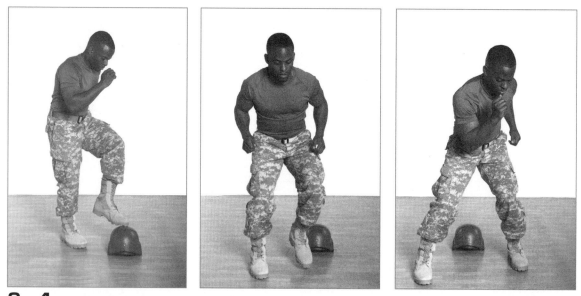

2-4 Quickly alternate your feet position 4 times, tapping the top of the helmet, then make a 360-degree shuffle around the helmet.

Repeat this drill in the opposite direction.

★ 360° BEAR CRAWL

This should be performed with body armor or a weighted vest.

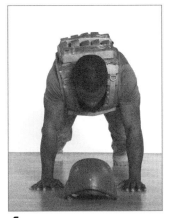

1 Start facedown on your hands and feet in front of a helmet on the ground.

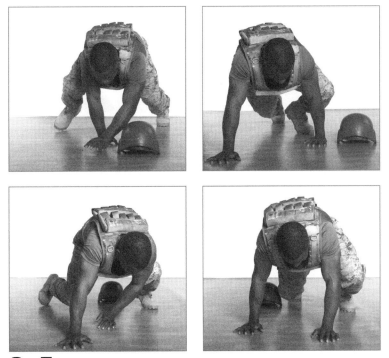

2-5 Keeping your knees off the ground and without crossing your hands or feet, quickly bear crawl in a 360-degree circle around the helmet.

Perform this drill in both directions.

★ OVER THE HILL

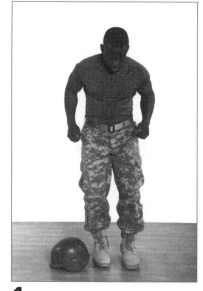

1 Start in the athletic position with your helmet on the ground outside your right foot.

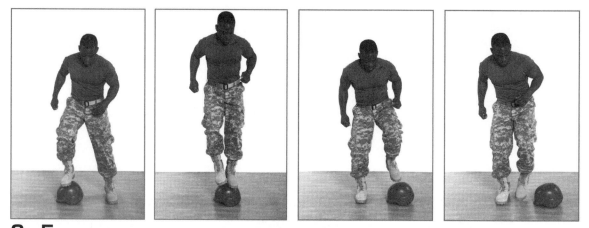

2-5 Without crossing your feet, step across to the opposite side of the helmet, left foot followed by the right foot.

Change direction as quickly as possible for the exercise duration.

★ SPRINT & TOUCH

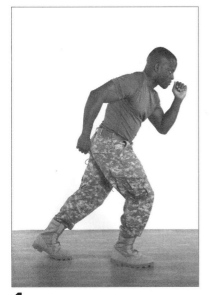 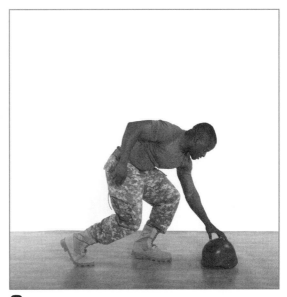

1 Sprint straight ahead to the desired distance in which your helmet is placed.

2 Once you reach the helmet, squat and touch the helmet.

Sprint back to the starting line.

★ SPRINT TO TOE TAP

1 Sprint straight ahead to the desired distance in which your helmet is placed.

2 Once you reach the helmet, perform your desired number of toe taps (page 126) for time or repetitions.

Sprint back to the starting line.

★ SPRINT TO 360° SHUFFLE

1 Sprint straight ahead to the desired distance in which your helmet is placed.

2 Once you reach the helmet, make a 360-degree shuffle (page 127) around the helmet.

Sprint back to the starting line.

★ JUMP TO SPRINT

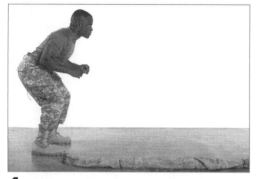

1 Start in the athletic position.

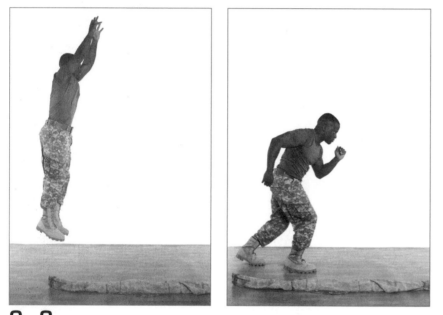

2-3 Perform 1 squat jump then quickly sprint to the opposite end of your combat uniform.

Once you reach the opposite end, perform another squat jump then quickly sprint back to the start position.

★ MARTIAL ARTS CARDIO ★

This section is designed to improve your cardio by performing a variety of martial arts strikes from karate, kickboxing and Muay Thai. When performed at maximum effort, this workout will kick your butt.

Make sure to familiarize yourself with the Fighter's Stance before you begin. The Fighter's Stance is your starting position for each striking technique.

FIGHTER'S STANCE

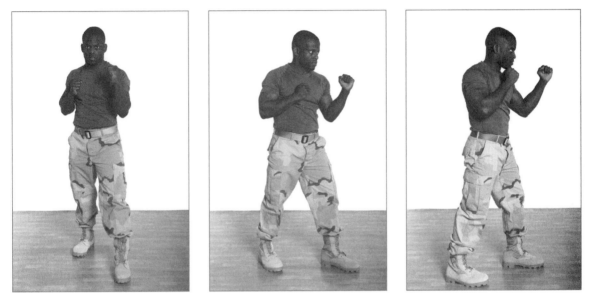

Stand with your dominant leg back, your knees slightly bent and your chin down, with your hands in a closed position by your chin.

★ JAB

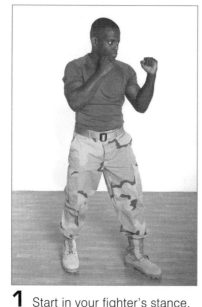

1 Start in your fighter's stance.

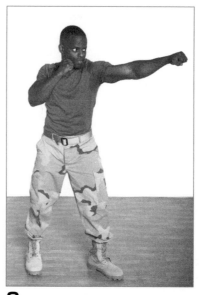

2 Drive your lead shoulder upward and fully extend your lead arm forward until your shoulder touches your chin. Your back hand should remain by your chin and be closed at all times.

Once your lead hand reaches full extension, quickly return to your fighter's stance.

★ CROSS

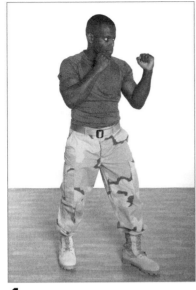

1 Start in your fighter's stance.

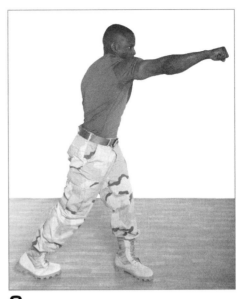

2 Slightly pivoting off your back foot, drive your rear shoulder upward and fully extend your back hand forward until your shoulder touches your chin. Your lead hand should remain by your chin and be closed at all times.

Once your rear hand reaches full extension, quickly return to your fighter's stance.

★ LEAD HOOK

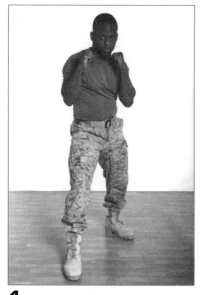

1 Start in your fighter's stance.

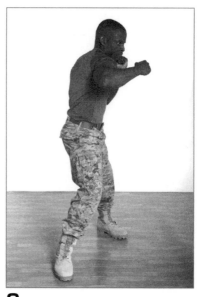

2 Fully rotate your torso, bringing your front hand, elbow and shoulder across your body along a half-circular path; they should all stay on the same horizontal plane. Shrug your lead shoulder in order to protect your jaw, and keep your back hand at your chin at all times.

Once your hook has been executed, quickly return to your fighter's stance.

★ LEAD-HAND UPPERCUT

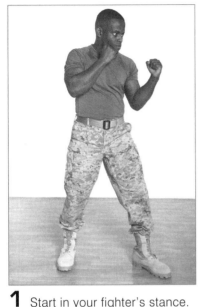

1 Start in your fighter's stance.

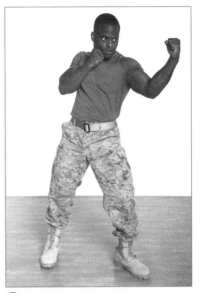

2 Drop your hips slightly downward, fully rotate your torso, shrug your front shoulder upward to your chin and extend your lead fist upward to approximately eye level.

Once your punch has been executed, quickly return to starting position.

★ REAR-HAND UPPERCUT

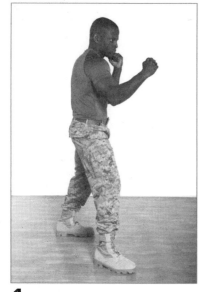

1 Start in your fighter's stance.

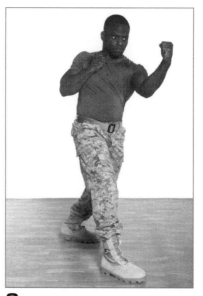

2 Drop your hips into a slightly downward position, fully rotate your torso, shrug your rear shoulder upward to your chin and extend your rear fist upward to approximately eye level.

Once your punch has been executed, quickly return to starting position.

★ LEAD ELBOW

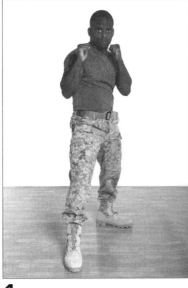

1 Start in your fighter's stance.

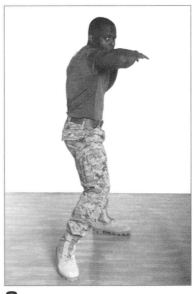

2 Swing your lead elbow upward, pulling your rear shoulder back. Rotate your hips and shoulders in a half-circular motion to generate striking power. Your elbow should not extend past your chin; your rear hand should always remain by your chin.

Once you perform the strike, quickly return to your fighter's stance.

★ REAR ELBOW

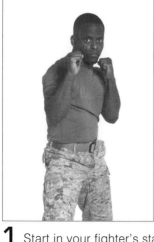

1 Start in your fighter's stance.

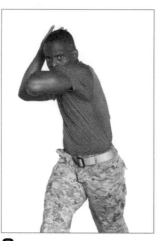

2 Swing your rear elbow upward, pulling your rear shoulder back. Rotate your hips and shoulders in a half-circular motion to generate striking power. Your elbow should not extend past your chin; your rear hand should always remain by your chin.

Once you perform the strike, quickly return to your fighter's stance.

★ DIP

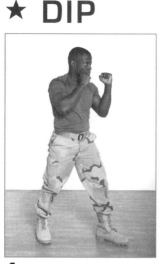

1 Start in your fighter's stance.

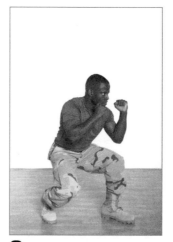

2 Keeping your hands by your chin, quickly squat to approximately 90 degrees.

Return to your fighter's stance.

★ FRONT KNEE

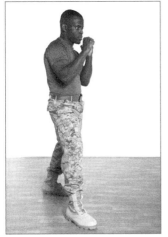

1 Start in your fighter's stance.

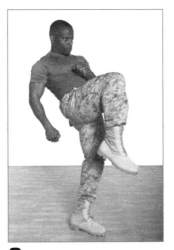

2 Maintaining a slight bend in your rear knee, drive your front knee forward while simultaneously pulling your hands to the outside of your front knee. Your toes should be pointed down when performing this strike.

★ REAR KNEE

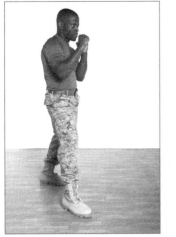

1 Start in your fighter's stance.

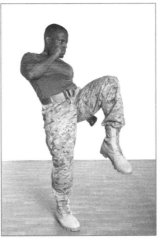

2 Maintaining a slight bend in your front knee, drive your rear knee forward while simultaneously pulling your rear hand to the outside of your lifted knee. Your toes should be pointed down when performing this strike.

★ PUSH KICK

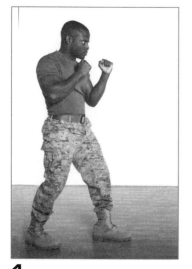

1 Start in your fighter's stance.

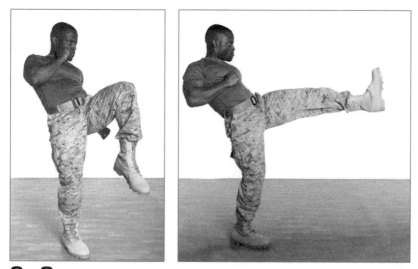

2-3 Lift your rear leg up and extend the leg with your toe pointed up. Dropping your rear hand down by your hip as you kick helps to generate extra kicking power.

★ SIDE KICK

This kick can be performed with the lead or rear leg.

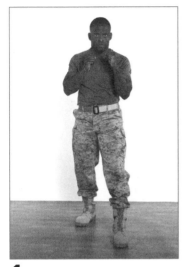

1 Start in your fighter's stance.

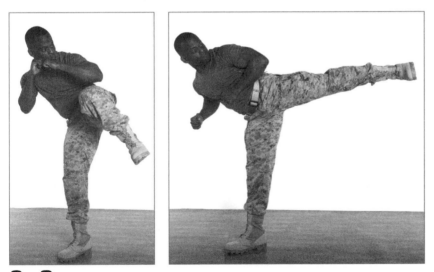

2-3 Shift your weight to your rear leg and, keeping your hands at your chin, tilt your upper body toward your rear leg. Lift your lead knee and extend your lead leg in a straight line, aiming with the heel of the foot. You're aiming your heel at an imaginary person's chest. As your hands drop, protect your chin with your lead shoulder.

Once you've executed the strike, quickly return to your fighter's stance.

20 PUNCHING & ELBOW COMBINATIONS

1 Jab, cross

2 Jab, jab, cross

3 Jab, cross, jab, cross

4 Jab, cross, hook

5 Cross, hook, cross

6 Cross, hook, rear-hand uppercut

7 Cross, lead elbow, cross

8 Lead-hand uppercut, dip, rear-hand uppercut

9 Lead elbow, rear elbow, lead-hand uppercut, rear-hand uppercut

10 Lead-hand uppercut, dip, hook, cross

11 Cross, lead elbow, cross, lead elbow

12 Dip, lead elbow, dip, rear elbow

13 Rear-hand uppercut, hook, cross

14 Hook, dip, hook, dip, hook

15 Hook, cross, dip, cross, dip, hook

16 Cross, lead-hand uppercut, dip, hook, cross, lead elbow

17 Jab, cross, hook, dip, dip, hook, cross, hook, cross

18 Hook, cross, lead-hand uppercut, cross, dip, cross

19 Rear elbow, hook, cross, lead elbow, cross, hook, hook

20 Freestyle (any combination)

20 PUNCHING & KICKING COMBINATIONS

1 Jab, cross, front kick

2 Jab, cross, lead knee, rear knee

3 Jab, hook, rear knee

4 Jab, front knee, lead front kick

5 Jab, lead front kick, rear front kick

6 Cross, hook, rear knee

7 Cross, cross, side kick

8 Cross, hook, rear knee, side kick

9 Cross, lead-hand uppercut, front knee, rear knee

10 Jab, cross, lead elbow, front knee, rear knee

11 Front knee, front knee, rear knee

12 Lead elbow, cross, front knee, front knee, front knee

13 Front knee, rear knee, front knee, rear knee

14 Front knee, side kick, front knee, side kick

15 Front knee, dip, rear knee, dip, side kick, side kick

16 Lead-hand uppercut, rear-hand uppercut, front knee, rear knee

17 Rear knee, side kick, rear knee, side kick

18 Dip, front knee, dip, rear knee

19 Dip, rear knee, rear front kick, dip, cross

20 Freestyle (any combination)

★ FLEXIBILITY ★

This section is designed to improve total-body flexibility. Improving your flexibility can increase your overall performance and decrease the chances of injury. Hold each stretch for approximately 10 seconds.

★ STANDING QUADRICEPS PULL

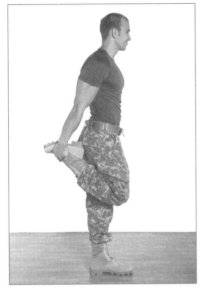

Stand and grab your right foot with your right hand. Maintain balance on your left leg. Hold for 10 seconds and then switch legs.

Muscles Stretched: Quadriceps (thigh)

★ ANKLE ROLLOUT

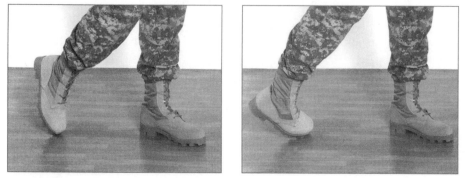

Stand with your right toe pointed into the ground and your right heel up. Gradually make small circles with your right foot in a clockwise and then counterclockwise direction. Perform approximately 10 seconds in each direction, and then switch legs.

Muscles Stretched: Outer leg, ligaments within the ankle

★ STANDING KNEE TO CHEST

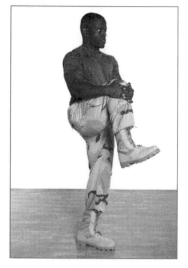

Stand and bring your right knee toward your chest. Place both hands around your knee or shin, holding the knee in position for 10 seconds before switching legs.

Muscles Stretched: Gluteus (buttocks), hamstrings, hip flexors

★ CALF STRETCH

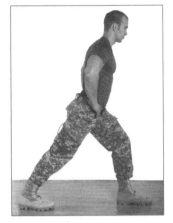

Start in a split lunge position with your hands on your hips; bend your front knee slightly and extend your back leg behind you with your heel on the ground. Constantly drive your back heel into the ground until you feel the stretch in your back leg. Hold for 10 seconds and then switch legs.

Muscles Stretched: Calf, outer shin, Achilles tendon

★ ACHILLES TENDON STRETCH

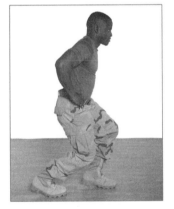

Start in a staggered stance with your hands on your hips; bend your front knee slightly and bend your back knee toward the ground, keeping your heel off the ground. Constantly drive your back knee toward the ground until you feel a stretch in your back leg and heel. Hold for 10 seconds and then switch legs.

Muscles Stretched: Outer shin, Achilles tendon

★ LATERAL LUNGE

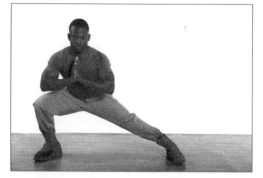

Stand with your feet shoulder-width apart and your hands together in prayer position. Keeping your feet flat on the ground at all times and legs straight, bend at your waist and lean toward your left leg. Sit your butt towards your heels as if you were performing a squat. Continue to push your butt back until you feel the stretch in your inner leg. Hold for 10 seconds and then switch legs.

Muscles Stretched: Groin, inner thigh, hamstrings

★ STRAIGHT-LEG STRETCH

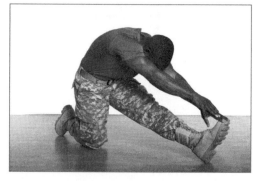

Place your right knee on the ground and your left leg fully extended in front of you with the left toes pointed up. Bend from the waist and reach toward your foot with one or both hands until you feel a stretch in the back of your left leg. Hold for 10 seconds and then switch legs.

Muscles Stretched: Gluteus (buttocks), hamstrings, calf, lower back

★ QUAD PULL

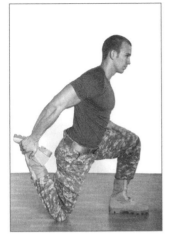

Sitting up on your knees, put your left foot flat on the ground in front of you so your left knee is at a 90-degree angle. Place your left hand on your left knee for balance as you reach behind you with your right hand to grasp your right foot. Pull your right foot in toward your right glute until you feel a stretch across the front of your right leg. Hold for 10 seconds and then switch legs.

Muscles Stretched: Quadriceps (thigh)

★ PRETZEL STRETCH

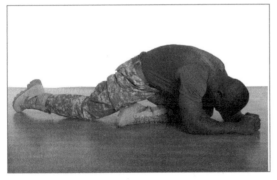

From kneeling, slide your right leg back and angle your left shin in front of you until you feel a stretch in your butt. Place your forearms on the ground in front of your left leg with your head looking down. Hold for 10 seconds and then switch legs.

Muscles Stretched: Gluteus (buttocks), hamstrings, groin, hips, lower back

★ GROIN STRETCH 1

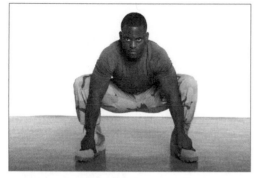

Stand with your feet slightly wider than your shoulders. Keeping your heels on the ground and your back straight, lower into a deep squat and place your elbows inside your knees. Push your knees out with your elbows until you feel a stretch in your inner thighs. Hold for 10 seconds.

Muscles Stretched: Groin

★ GROIN STRETCH 2

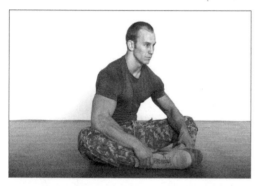

Sit on the ground with the bottoms of your shoes placed together. Grab the toes of your shoes and place your elbows on your inner thighs. Slowly push your thighs down with your elbows until you feel a stretch in your inner thighs. Hold for 10 seconds.

Muscles Stretched: Groin, hips, inner thigh

★ LOWER BACK STRETCH 1

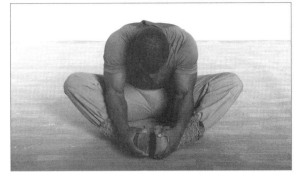

Sit on the ground with the bottoms of your shoes placed together and slightly move your feet away from your body. Grab the toes of your shoes and, as you exhale, slowly bring your forehead toward your feet. Hold for 10 seconds.

Muscles Stretched: Upper & lower back

★ LOWER BACK STRETCH 2

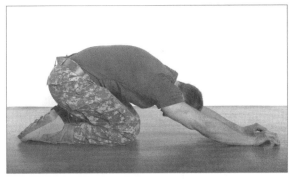

Kneel on the ground with your knees together and sit your butt back on your heels. Place your hands on the floor and reach forward until you feel a stretch in your back. Let your forehead release to the ground. Hold for 10 seconds.

Muscles Stretched: Upper & lower back

★ 3-POSITION STRETCH

Hold each position for 10 seconds.

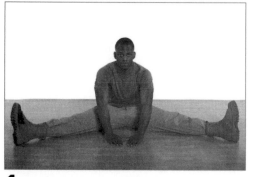

1 Sit on the ground with your legs wide apart and toes pointed upward.

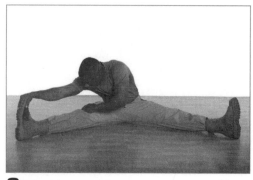

2 With your chest parallel to the ground, grab your right foot with your right hand to stretch your right leg.

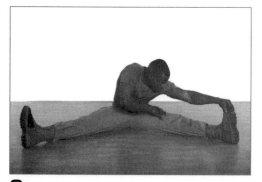

3 With your chest parallel to the ground, grab your left foot with your left hand to stretch your left leg.

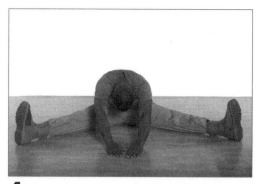

4 Reach to the middle with both hands and gradually lower yourself with each exhale.

Muscles Stretched: Groin, lower & upper back, hamstrings, hips, calf

★ HALF SPLIT

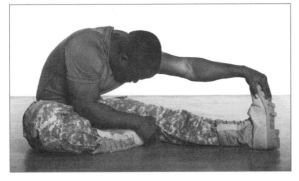

Sit on the ground with your left leg extended and your right foot placed on the inside of your inner left thigh. Take your left hand and grab the top of your left foot. Pull your chest toward your left knee each time you exhale until you feel a stretch. Hold for 10 seconds and then switch legs.

Muscles Stretched: Hamstrings, upper & lower back, calf

★ TWISTER

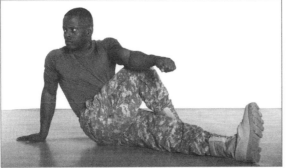

Sit on the ground with your left leg extended and your right foot placed to the outside of your left knee. Twist your upper body to the right and place your left elbow on the outside of your right knee. Place your right hand on the ground behind you to maintain balance. Hold for 10 seconds and then switch legs.

Muscles Stretched: Hips, back, sides

★ ASSISTED KNEE TO CHEST

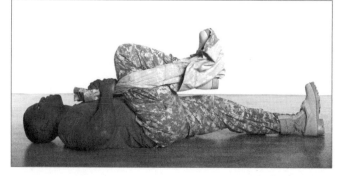

Lie on your back with your left leg extended. Wrap your combat uniform around your right foot and grab it with both hands. Slowly pull your right knee toward your chest until you feel a stretch. Hold for 10 seconds and then switch legs.

Muscles Stretched: Gluteus (buttocks), hamstrings, hip flexors

★ CROSS BODY

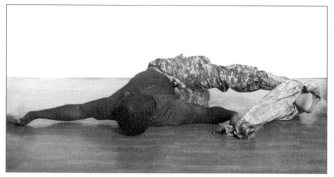

Lie on your back with your left arm and right leg extended. Place the combat uniform around your left foot and grab it with your right hand. Pull your left leg across your body in an upward motion. Hold for 10 seconds and then switch legs.

Muscles Stretched: Gluteus (buttocks), lower & upper back, hamstrings, hips, calf

★ STRAIGHT-LEG PULL

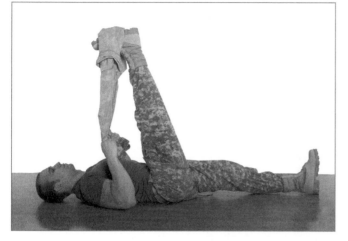

Lie on your back with your left leg extended and the combat uniform around your right foot. Grab the uniform with both hands and, keeping your leg straight, slowly pull your right leg toward your chest until you feel a stretch. Hold for 10 seconds and then switch legs.

Muscles Stretched: Gluteus (buttocks), hamstrings, calf

★ OPEN GATE

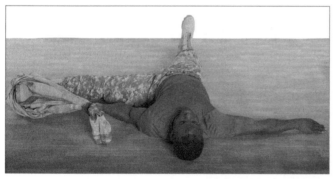

Lie on your back with your right arm and right leg extended. With your left hand, place the combat uniform around your left foot and pull your leg toward your head; keep your leg straight. Hold for 10 seconds and then switch legs.

Muscles Stretched: Gluteus (buttocks), groin, hamstrings, hips, calf

★ QUADRICEPS PULL

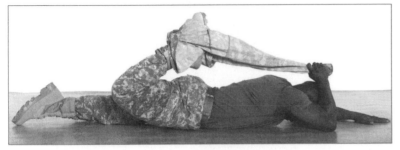

Lie on your stomach. With your right hand, place the combat uniform around your right foot and bend your right leg. Grab the uniform and pull your right leg toward your head until your right quad lifts off the ground. Hold for 10 seconds and then switch legs.

Muscles Stretched: Quadriceps (thigh), hips, lower back

★ ARM ACROSS

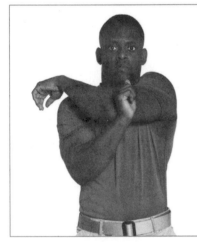 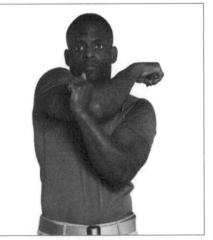

This stretch can be performed from a kneeling, sitting or standing position. Bring your left arm across your body and place your right hand behind your left elbow for support. Hold this position for 10 seconds and then switch arms.

Muscles Stretched: Triceps, deltoid, upper back

★ ARM BEHIND THE HEAD

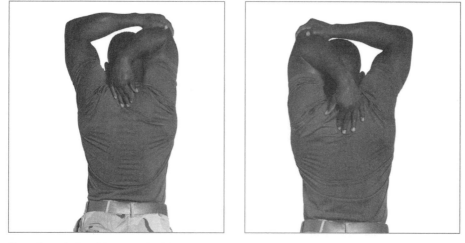

Stand or sit for this stretch. Move your right arm behind your head and place your right hand on the center of your back. Place your left hand on your right elbow and slowly apply downward pressure to your right elbow until you feel a stretch. Hold for 10 seconds and then switch arms.

Muscles Stretched: Triceps, deltoid, upper back

★ FLEXOR & EXTENSOR STRETCH

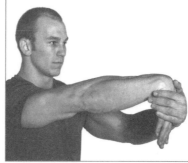

Stand with your feet shoulder-width apart and extend both arms in front of you with palms up. With your left hand, grab the fingertips of your right hand and slowly pull them towards your torso. Hold this position for 10 seconds and then switch hands.

Muscles Stretched: Forearm, hand ligaments

★ 4-WAY NECK STRETCH

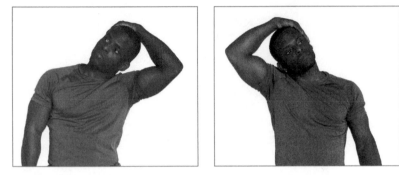

Stand with your feet shoulder-width apart and back straight. Reach
your left hand over your head and place it above your right ear.
Slowly pull your head toward your left shoulder until you feel a stretch
in your neck. Hold for 10 seconds and then switch sides.

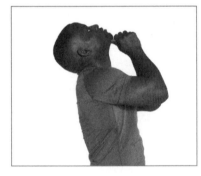

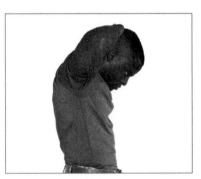

Stand with your feet shoulder-width apart and
back straight. Place your hands together with your
thumbs under your chin. Slowly push your head
backward until you feel a stretch in your neck.
Hold for 10 seconds.

Stand with your feet shoulder-width apart and
back straight. Lock your hands together and
place them behind your head. Slowly pull your
head forward until you feel a stretch in your neck.
Hold for 10 seconds.

Muscles Stretched: Neck

★ SIDE BEND

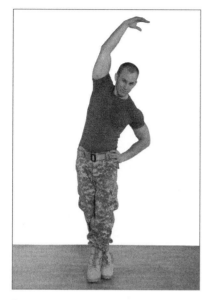

Stand and cross your right leg over your left leg. Place your left hand by your side and reach over your head to the left with your right hand. Hold for 10 seconds and then switch sides.

Muscles Stretched: Outer hips, upper back

★ ABDOMINAL STRETCH

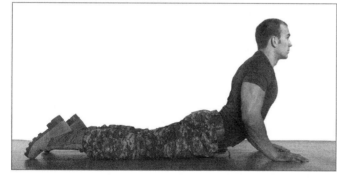

Lie on your stomach with your arms shoulder-width apart and palms flat on the ground. Push your torso up by extending your arms fully. Arch your back and press your hips to the ground. Hold for 10 seconds.

Muscles Stretched: Core (stomach muscles), hips, lower back

★ INDEX

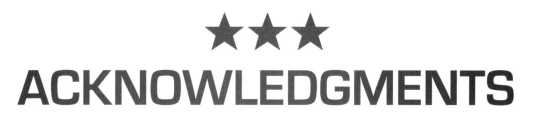

ACKNOWLEDGMENTS

First and foremost, I thank God for giving me the wisdom to create this program. Special thanks to all of the men and women of the military and First Response for all of your hard work, sacrifice and dedication, making this nation the best in the world! Lastly, I would like to thank Augusta Jr., Jamus, Belasco, Tommy Heffernan, and Dr. Creflo Dollar for always keeping me encouraged when I was discouraged.

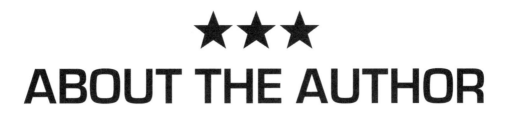

ABOUT THE AUTHOR

AUGUSTA DEJUAN HATHAWAY was born and raised in Murfreesboro, Tennessee. A graduate of Oakland High School in Murfreesboro, he served as captain of both the varsity football and track teams. As an adolescent, DeJuan was selected by his peers as Mr. Oakland, an honor bestowed upon the most physically fit high school male. As a collegiate student-athlete and captain of the football team at Maryville College (TN), DeJuan received his Bachelors of Arts in physical education in 2005.

Upon graduating, he served as a strength coach with the University of Hawaii-Manoa's athletic program and received his Master's degree in kinesiology (2009). After completing his Master's, he served as the fitness coordinator for the U.S. Navy and Marine Corps at Kaneohe Marine Base—Hawaii. During his tenure, he received a Civilian Appreciation Award for his impact on overall solider fitness. DeJuan also presented his fitness program to Navy and Marine personnel at the 2009 Rim of the Pacific Exercise (RIMPAC). DeJuan also served as a strength and conditioning specialist at Ft. Benning, Georgia, from 2011–2013. During his tenure, he was honored with awards such as Commanding General's Award of Excellence, Commander's Award for Public Service, and Support Cadre of the Cycle on two occasions for his extraordinary work in strength and conditioning, improving the physical fitness of military personnel.

DeJuan currently serves as a strength and conditioning specialist for the U.S. Special Operational Forces at Ft. Bragg, North Carolina. He has also served at prestigious programs such as those at the University of Tennessee, University of Nebraska and Hawaii Pacific University. DeJuan is a certified strength and conditioning specialist through the National Strength and Conditioning Association (NSCA) and strength and conditioning coach certified through the Collegiate Strength and Conditioning Coaches Association (CSCCa). He is also a Level 1 and Level 2 certified in Army Combatives. When not conditioning soldiers for combat, DeJuan is a professional mixed martial artist who remains undefeated. For more information about him, visit hathawayfitness.com.